KNOWLEDGE MANAGEMENT
in PUBLIC HEALTH

KNOWLEDGE MANAGEMENT
in PUBLIC HEALTH

Edited by
Jay Liebowitz
Richard A. Schieber
Joanne D. Andreadis

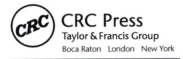

CRC Press
Taylor & Francis Group
Boca Raton   London   New York

CRC Press is an imprint of the
Taylor & Francis Group, an **informa** business

CRC Press
Taylor & Francis Group
6000 Broken Sound Parkway NW, Suite 300
Boca Raton, FL 33487-2742

© 2010 by Taylor and Francis Group, LLC
CRC Press is an imprint of Taylor & Francis Group, an Informa business

No claim to original U.S. Government works

Printed in the United States of America on acid-free paper
10 9 8 7 6 5 4 3 2 1

International Standard Book Number: 978-1-4398-0600-5 (Hardback)

Library of Congress Cataloging-in-Publication Data

Knowledge management in public health / editors, Jay Liebowitz, Richard A. Schieber, Joanne Andreadis.
        p. ; cm.
    Includes bibliographical references and index.
    ISBN 978-1-4398-0600-5 (hardcover : alk. paper)
    1. Knowledge management. 2. Public health. 3. Medical informatics. I. Liebowitz, Jay. II. Schieber, Richard A. III. Andreadis, Joanne. IV. Title.
    [DNLM: 1. Public Health Informatics. 2. Information Management. WA 26.5 K73 2010]

    R858.A3K56 2010
    362.1068--dc22   2009021574

Visit the Taylor & Francis Web site at
http://www.taylorandfrancis.com

and the CRC Press Web site at
http://www.crcpress.com

Dedication

Dedicated to all people striving to make a difference in the world.

To those public health professionals, educators, and students who tirelessly serve for the greater good.

To Janet, Jason, and Kenny—I'm so lucky!

To my mother, my husband Oliver, and my children, Alexandra and Christopher.

Contents

Foreword

According to Wikipedia, knowledge management (KM) comprises a range of practices used in an organization to identify, create, represent, distribute, and enable adoption of insights and experiences. What's different about this when compared with business as usual? For one thing, I am citing Wikipedia, rather than an international authority, book, or published manuscript. Wikipedia is a form of knowledge convergence put into an electronic document with the full expectation that it will mutate to contain more and better information by any number of experts and thinkers as the topic matures. It is an electronic expression of Darwinian forces, an open book whose last page will never be written. And as such, wikis are a manifestation of KM processes. Wikipedia lies within and is accessed through the Internet, an electronic entity that is itself a manifestation of communal knowledge.

The concept of a wiki is not new, but its electronic format is enormously more efficient. In the spring of 1900, archaeological tablets written in Linear B, an ancient script form of the Mycenaean language, were excavated at Knossos in Crete. Scholars of classical Greece were unable to decipher the language, so the thinking at that time was that these tablets were not written in Greek. For years the tablets remained undeciphered. After World War II, a British architect and classical scholar, Michael Ventris, became interested in the mystery. Perhaps most importantly, he shared the information with a group of people he thought would be most likely to shed light on the mystery. He asked for their insights and shared their responses, repeating the process often. It was similar to Wikipedia before the electronic possibility. This example of KM led Ventris to solve the mystery. He managed to combine the knowledge and hunches of a group. More recently, Dr. Jeffery Koplan at Emory University has used the Internet to get many people to consider the definition of the term "global health." What was extraordinary a half-century ago has become a daily occurrence in problem solving today, in part due to the enormous increase in efficiency rendered by computers and information technology, and in part because of the need to better understand our increasingly complex world.

KM has the goal of synthesizing old and new information to create sensible solutions. It attempts to do so by compiling written, spoken, and thought knowledge into electronic document formats so that it is available, readable, searchable, and helpful to others. Such information is either explicit (written) or tacit (thought, and therefore accessible only to that individual). Unwritten, or tacit, knowledge often is difficult to obtain and incorporate into other knowledge already written. In recent years, it became clear that the archives on smallpox eradication are deficient to tell the story of that effort. In an attempt to make tacit knowledge explicit, Dr. David Sencer has headed up a project to extract oral histories from the participants of the eradication program.

In addition to the translation of pertinent tacit knowledge into writing, KM activities include a perpetual effort to compile explicit knowledge germane to a problem so that it may come to bear on that problem. While its definition is conceptual, KM is best known by the tools it creates to join experts together to create new knowledge. These tools include expertise locators such as institutional white pages; collaborative technologies such as Lotus Notes, blogs, wikis, and social networks such as Facebook or MySpace; communities of practice where experts and those interested in a particular area can meet virtually to discuss aspects and applications of the field; the underlying aspects of information technology needed to create and maintain these functions; and other mechanisms. Some aspects, such as the Linear B example, predate the early development of modern KM systems (circa 1995), but had a similar purpose. Some tools may already be in place in a public health organization. For example, e-mail has consistently provided a solid way to communicate policy decisions, and the information and data that led to their creation. Where KM differs is the expectation that many people at many levels will participate in the development of a new policy, and a place will be made available for a healthy discussion and record of its pros and cons. The capacity of such systems to allow the search for prior experience cannot be overstated. This search capability quite often obviates the need for one-to-one telephone communication, and makes use of archival information that may have preceded the current decision maker. The smallpox example suggests that organizations should establish a better way of capturing and recording implicit and tacit historical and current events, along with the opinions and beliefs, policies, programs, and their outcomes, in real time whenever possible.

How can KM improve public health actions? One of the principal assets of public health departments, perhaps the chief one, is the development and distribution of usable knowledge. The most important medical advance in the twentieth century may be that ordinary people were able to use science, even if they were not scientists themselves. The improvement of health over the past century resulted from millions of daily decisions on exercising, food choices, smoking, and use of seat belts, helmets, insulin, vitamins, blood pressure medication, anticoagulants, vaccines, sun screens, etc. It involved making scientific knowledge available for individuals in a usable way and sometimes through laws imposed on everyone. Therefore, public health units, whether federal, state, or local in scope, need to ensure that the knowledge they provide is current, user-friendly, engaging, accurate, and representative of both the majority and less popular opinions. The tools of KM—especially blogs, wikis, and document-sharing management and control—can be of benefit in ensuring that these requirements are met with the least difficulty and accessible by all. KM is not truth, but it is a system for seeking truth.

KM can help public health maximize the efficiency of staff. It provides a technological solution with a profound database. Practitioners can develop sound policies in less time in response to a new problem when they have something akin to Google for Public Health that provides the information he or she needs, and a blog whose discussion threads can help determine what such information means. This could lead to a rapidly developed but well-considered policy that is data-driven and benefits from, in a sense, the wisdom of the crowd.

What would be the chief barriers to engaging in such activities? The usual responses would be the lack of resources—personnel or funds—to begin developing such a system. The fault in logic here is the same logic error made when people say they do not have resources for prevention, which, if in place, could likely reduce the need for such resources. The KM system is exactly what is needed to save resources, and will likely reduce dependence on a large number of personnel to research and understand a problem.

Another barrier to engagement is unfamiliarity with such systems. Although there is a substantial amount of information already available electronically on the Web, much of it is unsorted, in various formats, and speaks to different audiences. A value of this book is to help the reader become familiar with the many elements of KM while understanding how to start such a system in his or her own work environment. I emphasize "start" because with the relatively few resources likely to be made available to develop it, a full-blown KM program will take time and energy. The first few chapters of this book describe why and how to build such a system, while the other chapters give specific examples describing the development and value added of such a system in a variety of public health environments.

Tough or quick decision making has always benefitted enormously from well-considered knowledge based on the maximum amount of pertinent information available at the time—this has not changed. What is new in our present public health environment is the need to do this more often and with fewer personnel available relative to the services expected by the public. Better use of information under a KM system is well-suited to serve that master.

William H. Foege, MD, MPH
Senior Fellow, Global Health Program
Bill and Melinda Gates Foundation

Preface

Reversing the Knowledge Paradigm

Starting Early

A paradox exists as many knowledge-centered students move into their public health and medical school studies where mentoring and apprenticeship programs are the rule, not the exception. Whether shadowing physicians or working in clinical care or applied public health teams, collaboration is a fundamental critical success factor for today's health care professional.[1,2,3,8] A knowledge-sharing culture becomes the norm rather than the isolated case. Thus, a paradox exists when these students whose "knowledge is power" attitudes have thrived must now adapt and assimilate to a "*sharing* knowledge is power" philosophy. We must start early in the undergraduate careers of future public health and health care professionals. How can this transformation easily take place in order to better prepare future doctors and public health professionals?

The simple answer is through the field of knowledge management. Knowledge management focuses on improving collaboration, knowledge flows, and communication.[4,6,7] It looks at how best to leverage knowledge internally and externally, and is a process for creating value from the intellectual assets. Knowledge management typically involves the iterative cycle of knowledge identification and capture, knowledge sharing, knowledge application, and knowledge creation. Knowledge management can serve as the integrative mechanism to form bridges across the isolated islands of knowledge. Those pursuing knowledge management have found that innovation and creativity are often increased, a sense of community and belonging is enhanced, and the institutional memory is further preserved.

How can these concepts then apply to preparing our students for their forthcoming public health and medical school educations? This can be done from both a codification, systems-oriented "collection" approach and a personalization "connection" approach. Orientation programs and team-building exercises can help foster greater connections for public health and premedical students. Creating online communities, people locator systems, and group pages for teamwork and discussion forums also will encourage collaboration to take place. Today's student is already used to social networking sites, such as Facebook, YouTube, MySpace, and others, so the Generation Yers are already very adept at "building bridges."[5] Also, integrating various issues into the classroom that span across a discipline's boundaries will help students to analyze problems from a multidisciplinary, synergistic perspective versus through a myopic lens.

Mentoring also can be used effectively to facilitate knowledge exchange and knowledge retention. Of course, the Pre-Health Professional Advising Office and the Pre-Health Honor Society in most universities provide wonderful guidance in a mentoring-type role. The Student Doctor Network (http://www.studentdoctor .net) also provides a mechanism for exchanging ideas and experiences in preparing for a medical profession.

Separate from a frequently asked questions list, it may be helpful to have a lessons learned and best practice system in order to formally document dos and don'ts relating to premedical and public health studies, medical-related research, physician shadowing, interviewing, volunteering, medical school selection, and other related premed and public health areas. Different from online communities, a lessons learned and best practice system has the success and failure tips formally vetted before acceptance into the lessons learned system. The Pre-Health Professional Advising Office, for example, may serve as the committee that would include selected students, faculty, alumni, and staff to meet every month to review the submitted lessons learned for possible inclusion in the lessons learned system. The lessons learned system would allow users to learn from others' experiences, as well as serve as a formal repository for building this institutional memory. This system should also include a user profiling feature, through which users can indicate which areas they are interested in receiving lessons. As a new lesson is entered into the system that fits the user's profile, the user will automatically be sent an e-mail with the URL to access that new lesson. In this manner, the "push" approach (versus the "pull" approach) will provide a more active method for people to receive appropriate lessons.

Another interesting approach borrowed from the knowledge management community for educating our premedical and public health students could be to have team-taught courses with professors from different backgrounds. For example, it may be beneficial to have an instructor-led team of business, bioethics, technology, science, history, and public health professors to integrate and infuse these various topics within the traditional premed curriculum. Instead of covering them in separate modules, various issues that touch on these areas may be posed, which would then have to be discussed, researched, and solved by the students. In this case, the professor may serve as the facilitator, adviser, or coach versus the usual knowledge provider role. This approach has worked quite well in integrated science and technology programs such as at James Madison University, for example.

As medical errors could result from miscommunication and poor handoffs between health care individuals and teams, knowledge management principles can be applied early on in the future doctor and public health professional's educational experience to assuage these possible risks. By capitalizing on the talents and social networking skills of our undergraduates, collaboration and communication can be further enhanced by incorporating knowledge management concepts and applications in the classroom. Those approaches, as discussed in this Preface, may provoke others to explore integrative mechanisms for building synergy among the public health and premedical student communities. By doing so, our future health care professionals will be better prepared to handle the complexities of both their professional and personal lives.

The Way Ahead

The impetus for this book was to expose public health and health care practitioners, students, and educators to the idea of applying knowledge management in their professional and everyday lives. This book is one of the first volumes, if not *the* first, on knowledge management in public health. The chapters are written by some of the leading individuals and organizations involved in applying knowledge management in public health worldwide. We thank them for their valuable contributions to the book. We are grateful for the encouraging words written by Dr. Foege in the Foreword. We also owe our appreciation to John Wyzalek, Tara Nieuwesteeg, and the entire Taylor & Francis staff for their help in publishing this book. We hope that you have as much fun reading the book as we did in putting it together. Enjoy!

Dr. Jay Liebowitz
Dr. Richard A. Schieber
Dr. Joanne D. Andreadis

References

1. Dawes, M. and U. Sampson. 2003. Knowledge management in clinical practice: A systematic review of information seeking behavior in physicians. *International Journal of Medical Informatics* 71(1).
2. De Lusignan, S., K. Pritchard, and T. Chan. 2002. A knowledge management model for clinical practice. *Journal of Postgraduate Medicine* 48(4).
3. Kommalage, M. and S. Gunawardena. 2008. Feasibility of introducing information technology-based activities into medical curricula in developing countries. *Medical Education Journal* 42(1, January).
4. Liebowitz, J. 2006. *What They Didn't Tell You About Knowledge Management.* Lanham, MD: Scarecrow Press/Rowman & Littlefield.
5. Liebowitz, J. 2007. *Social Networking: The Essence of Innovation.* Lanham, MD: Scarecrow Press/Rowman & Littlefield.

6. Liebowitz, J., ed. 2008. *Making Cents Out of Knowledge Management.* Lanham, MD: Scarecrow Press/Rowman & Littlefield.
7. Liebowitz, J. 2006. *Strategic Intelligence: Business Intelligence, Competitive Intelligence, and Knowledge Management.* New York: Auerbach Publishing/Taylor & Francis.
8. Liebowitz, J. and J. Liebowitz. 2006. Trends and management challenges of the changing workforce: Knowledge management as a possible remedy. *LabMedicine,* June.

Editors

Dr. Jay Liebowitz is a professor in the Carey Business School at Johns Hopkins University. He was recently ranked as one of the top ten knowledge management researchers/practitioners out of 11,000 worldwide. He is the program director of the Graduate Certificate in Competitive Intelligence at Johns Hopkins University and the MS-ITS Capstone Director. He is founder and editor-in-chief of *Expert Systems with Applications: An International Journal*, published by Elsevier. Previously, Dr. Liebowitz was the first knowledge management officer at the NASA Goddard Space Flight Center; the Robert W. Deutsch Distinguished Professor of Information Systems at the University of Maryland, Baltimore County; chair of Artificial Intelligence at the U.S. Army War College; and professor of management science at George Washington University. Dr. Liebowitz was a Fulbright Scholar, is an IEEE-USA Federal Communications Commission Executive Fellow, and was the Computer Educator of the Year of the International Association for Computer Information Systems. He has consulted and lectured worldwide and can be reached at jliebow1@jhu.edu.

Dr. Richard A. Schieber is a pediatrician and a medical epidemiologist at the Centers for Disease Control and Prevention in Atlanta. Dr. Schieber is board certified in general pediatrics, pediatric cardiology, and pediatric critical care medicine. He has experience working in university practice, private practice, federal government, county public health department, and injury advocacy groups. In the 1980s he began the Pediatric Critical Care Medicine Division at Emory University and served as its first division director and medical director of the pediatric intensive care unit. In 1992, he left full-time clinical practice and moved to the CDC, where he has served public health as an epidemiologist in many capacities—childhood injury prevention, adverse cardiac events following smallpox vaccination, immunizations—and also as the first senior advisor for Pandemic Influenza in 2005–2006. Since October 2007 he has been the senior medical adviser for a new program that blends situation awareness and knowledge management at the CDC.

Dr. Joanne D. Andreadis leads the CDC's Innovation Team in the Office of Strategy and Innovation, office of the director, at the Centers for Disease Control and Prevention in Atlanta, Georgia. Dr. Andreadis's focus is to encourage entrepreneurial research and systems-based solutions to public health challenges by fostering a culture of innovation, promoting exploration of new approaches that translate science into action, and fostering open innovation to accelerate public health impact. Dr. Andreadis has more than twenty-six years of experience as a bench scientist and with numerous publications. Prior to her current position, Dr. Andreadis was the chief of the Botulism Public Health Research and Preparedness Unit in the National Center for Zoonotic, Vector-Borne, and Enteric Diseases. The focus of her group was to identify gaps in public health laboratory response capability, to work with cross-sector partners to develop innovative solutions, and to transition novel capabilities to national and international public health laboratories. Before starting at the CDC, Joanne was a principal investigator at the Center for Bio/Molecular Science and Engineering at the U.S. Naval Research Laboratory, a corporate research laboratory for the Navy and Marine Corps in Washington, D.C. Her work there involved developing methods to support the production of artificial biological polymers, developing tissue-based biological sensors for biothreat detection, and developing high throughput multivariate tests for identification, subtyping, and profiling of target organisms. Dr. Andreadis was a National Research Council Postdoctoral Fellow and received her doctorate in biochemistry and molecular biology at the University of Maryland.

List of Contributors

Joanne D. Andreadis
Office of Strategy and Innovation
Centers for Disease Control and
    Prevention
Atlanta, Georgia

Debra Bara
Public Health Informatics Institute
Decatur, Georgia

Laura Birx
Nutrition Division, U.S. Agency for
    International Development
Washington, D.C.

Paul F. Bugni
myPublicHealth Knowledge
    Management Group
Center for Public Health Informatics
School of Public Health and
    Community Medicine
University of Washington
Seattle, Washington

Masud Cader
International Finance Corp.
The World Bank Group
Carey Business School
Johns Hopkins University
Baltimore, Maryland

Liz Dahlstrom
myPublicHealth Knowledge
    Management Group
Center for Public Health Informatics
School of Public Health
    and Community Medicine
University of Washington
Seattle, Washington

Kara DeCorby
McMaster University
Hamilton, Ontario, Canada

Neha Desai
Knowledge and Information Services
Association of Public Health Laboratories
Silver Spring, Maryland

Maureen Dobbins
School of Nursing
McMaster University
Hamilton, Ontario, Canada

Sterling Elliott
Association of State and Territorial
    Health Officials
Arlington, Virginia

Angela M. Fix
Association of State and Territorial
  Health Officials
Arlington, Virginia

Sherrilynne S. Fuller
myPublicHealth Knowledge
  Management Group
Center for Public Health Informatics
School of Public Health and
  Community Medicine
University of Washington
Seattle, Washington

Lori Greco
McMaster University
Hamilton, Ontario, Canada

Heather Husson
McMaster University
Hamilton, Ontario, Canada

Richard Iams
Knowledge Management Practice
Project Performance Corp.
McLean, Virginia

Emil Ivanov
Carey Business School
Johns Hopkins University
Baltimore, Maryland

Edwin Lee
McMaster University
Hamilton, Ontario, Canada

Jay Liebowitz
Carey Business School
Johns Hopkins University
Baltimore, Maryland

Arthur J. Murray
Applied Knowledge Sciences Inc.
The George Washington University
  Institute for Knowledge and
  Innovation
Boyce, Virginia

Robert Rej
Wadsworth Center for Laboratories
  and Research
New York State Department of Health
Albany, New York
and
Knowledge Management Committee
Association of Public Health
  Laboratories
Silver Spring, Maryland

Debra Revere
Global Partners in Public Health
  Informatics
myPublicHealth Knowledge
  Management Group
Center for Public Health Informatics
School of Public Health and
  Community Medicine
University of Washington
Seattle, Washington

Patricia Ringers
Organizational Development
  Consultant
Severna Park, Maryland

Paula Robeson
Health Evidence
School of Nursing
McMaster University
Hamilton, Ontario, Canada

Richard A. Schieber
Public Health Service
BioPHusion Program
Office of Critical Information
    Integration and Exchange
National Center for Zoonotic, Vector-
    Borne, and Enteric Diseases
Centers for Disease Control and
    Prevention
Atlanta, Georgia

Irene Stephens
Association of State and Territorial
    Health Officials
Arlington, Virginia

Daiva Trillis
McMaster University
Hamilton, Ontario, Canada

Richard Van West-Charles
Pan American Health Organization
World Health Organization
Washington, D.C.

Ellen Wild
Public Health Informatics Institute
Decatur, Georgia

KNOWLEDGE MANAGEMENT

I

Today and Beyond

Chapter 1

The Quick Basics of Knowledge Management

Jay Liebowitz

Contents

Introduction

Knowledge management may seem like a mysterious term to many, but its roots are deeply entrenched in a variety of disciplines, including organizational behavior, human resources management, information technology, cognitive psychology, anthropology, sociology, education, and others. Knowledge management refers to how best to leverage knowledge internally and externally. In other words, it deals with creating a process for generating value-added benefits from an organization's intellectual assets. Even though the term was coined in the early 1980s, the underlying principles really weren't adequately conveyed until the mid-1990s when Web-based and intranet technologies were becoming more commonplace in organizations. These technologies enabled the bridges to be built across the isolated islands of knowledge

3

often siloed in organizations. However, even before these enabling technologies existed, knowledge management had been done for eons, especially considering the use of storytelling as a means for sharing and transferring knowledge.

Even though the definition of knowledge management may not be universal, many organizations engage in knowledge management for a variety of reasons. The primary ones typically include: increasing innovation, better organizing the corporate knowledge, building the institutional memory of the firm, creating a stronger sense of community and belonging, and providing a better mechanism for learning from others. The hope is that knowledge management leads to knowledge creation and discovery, which can ultimately be translated into the creation of new ideas, products, or services.

Most people will agree that knowledge management has four key processes: knowledge identification and capture, knowledge sharing, knowledge application, and knowledge creation. Important knowledge is typically captured, then exchanged with others, applied in various contexts, and then used to generate new knowledge. Once knowledge is generated, it goes through the iterative cycle of being captured, shared, and applied. Of course, not all knowledge may be important enough to be captured as part of the living memory of the organization. Thus, a vetting process may have to be conducted to determine the various types of knowledge that should be captured. These may include subject-matter-domain knowledge, strategic knowledge, relationship knowledge (who knows whom), process knowledge, general knowledge, historical knowledge, and others. Also, some knowledge may be strategic to the mission and vision of the organization five years or more into the future, whereas other types of knowledge may be more tactical but may be a critical part of getting things done.

In looking at knowledge management, most practitioners believe there are three main components of knowledge management: people/culture, process, and technology. Many will say that 80 percent of knowledge management is the people/culture and process components, with the other 20 percent being technology. Technology serves as an enabling mechanism for knowledge management, but the real difficulty lies more in the other two components.

The people/culture component refers to building and nurturing a knowledge-sharing culture. That is, how do you transform a culture into a knowledge-sharing one, versus perhaps a knowledge-hoarding environment? Making the paradigm shift from a "knowledge is power" adage to a "sharing knowledge is power" philosophy may not be as easy as it sounds. Linking the recognition and reward system to learning and knowledge-sharing behaviors may help encourage knowledge sharing to take place. More important is building interpersonal trust so that others feel comfortable in sharing.

The process component of knowledge management is equally as critical as the people/culture side. Seamlessly embedding knowledge management processes into one's daily work life is essential so that people don't become burdened with yet one more thing to do. Incorporating the capture and retrieval of lessons learned as part of a project team's development life cycle is an example of a knowledge management process that can be embedded within each project management team. Having a brown-bag "lunch-and-learn" session with others to report back on a conference trip and engage in some discussions may be another example. Receiving daily industry news and reports that are important to your work through the knowledge management system may be a way to further hook people. People shouldn't have to feel that knowledge management is another thing to do on top of an already full plate.

Technology can facilitate the creation of a unified knowledge network in order to integrate across the functional stovepipes in many organizations. Trying to create a "push" approach versus a "pull" approach can be accomplished through technology. For example, creating a user-profiling agent to determine the areas of interest an individual is working on during a set month can be used as a proactive way to disseminate new lessons that may match a user's interest profile. This is an example of a push approach, whereby a URL link to new lessons that fit the user's interests are sent to the user via e-mail, instead of the pull (passive) approach of the user searching a lessons-learned database for appropriate lessons of interest. Aside from lessons-learned systems, technology can be used to support online communities, blogs, wikis, expertise-locator systems, document management systems, social-networking maps, and the like.

With the three knowledge management components in mind—people/culture, process, and technology—most people favor a codification or personalization approach to knowledge management, although both will be applied with one taking dominance. The codification approach is a more systems-oriented technique that has a technology-based orientation. Its focus is more on the "collection" side of knowledge management versus the "connection" personalization side. The personalization approach favors the people-to-people connection. However, there is a gray area between both approaches as, for example, online communities, blogs, and expertise-locator systems encourage the connection and sharing of ideas between people but certainly have a technology component in terms of providing the software to make these media possible. The key with the codification or personalization approach is that the organization should apply the most natural approach that fits its culture. For example, if many people are technologists and scientists and perhaps may be slightly introverted in nature, they may prefer the systems-oriented, codification approach because they already feel comfortable working in a systems environment. Other organizations that may be more team-based, high-energy, and extroverted may prefer to apply a personalization approach, such as formal mentoring programs, job shadowing, job rotations, onboarding, coaching, and the like. By aligning the knowledge management approach with the organizational culture, there may be greater acceptance of the knowledge management techniques being put in place.

Besides alignment with the organizational culture, the knowledge management strategy must be aligned with the strategic mission and vision of the organization. If there is misalignment here, the knowledge management approach will be suboptimized and may fall into nonuse. Those knowledge management efforts typically fail due to the incongruence between the organization's strategic plan and objectives and the knowledge management strategy created. In other cases, knowledge management initiatives may fail due to a poorly designed knowledge management plan.

In providing a holistic view of the organization, knowledge management should be part of the organization's overarching human capital strategy. The human capital strategy looks at attracting and developing the organization's workforce of the future to meet the strategic mission and vision. As such, the "owner" of the human capital strategy is typically the chief human capital officer, chief learning officer, or the like. There should be four main pillars of a human capital strategy: competency management, performance management, knowledge management, and change management. Competency management deals with determining and developing the competencies needed in the organization's current and future workforce. Performance management provides a mechanism for rewarding people for achieving the desired levels of proficiencies and competencies, as well as possibly providing negative incentives for those who don't. Knowledge management, as we have been discussing, deals with how best to leverage knowledge internally and externally. Change management relates to the kinds of organizational culture and business process changes that need to be made so the human capital strategy can be successful. These four pillars serve as the foundation for the organization's human capital strategy.

As related to knowledge management, organizations typically progress through five maturity levels in their knowledge management journeys. The first level, zero, is "nonawareness," whereby the organization has not heard of knowledge management. Level 1 is "awareness," in which the organization is introduced to knowledge management and knowledge sharing concepts. Level 2 is "initiation," where small knowledge-management pilots are developed and sprinkled throughout the organization. Level 3 is "intrigue and interest," whereby the knowledge management pilots spark enthusiasm and interest and give way to full-blown knowledge management projects. Level 4 is "penetration," whereby the discovery phase leads to mass appeal, and employees are embracing knowledge sharing tenets, as well as embedding knowledge management activities into their daily working lives. Level 5 is "utility," whereby nirvana is created through the knowledge management activities, and the organization (and its people) realizes the collective value of knowledge sharing and can assess the utility and resulting impact of knowledge management on the organization.

In the authors' experience, we have found that most of the organizations are somewhere between Level 0 through Level 3, and very few are at Level 4 or Level 5. Some organizations, such as The Aerospace Corporation, are very mature in terms of their knowledge retention strategy. Knowledge retention deals with how best to retain the knowledge of people before they leave the organization, as well as leveraging their knowledge between projects. The Aerospace Corporation was selected as a Best-Practice organization by APQC (http://www.apqc.org) for its knowledge retention and knowledge management activities. In its March 2008 benchmarking report, "Retaining Today's Knowledge for Tomorrow's Work Force," APQC mentions some of its key findings (http://www.apqc.org/portal/apqc/ksn?paf_gear_id=contentgearhome&paf_dm =full&pageselect=detail&docid=149923):

- Communities of practice are a primary vehicle to identify, capture, and transfer knowledge.
- Best-practice organizations apply facilitated knowledge transfer approaches—such as knowledge audits, handoff documents, lessons learned, and interviews—to capture job-related knowledge.
- Mentoring and apprenticeship programs play a key role in tacit knowledge transfer.
- Best-practice organizations engage with subject matter experts in a formal, structured manner for the purposes of knowledge retention and transfer.
- Storytelling continues to play an important role in imparting history, context, heroes, and values to employees.
- In-house training organizations are taking on a larger, more strategic role with regard to knowledge retention and transfer.
- Knowledge retention and transfer approaches span the employment life cycle, and best-in-class organizations continue to tap the expertise of retirees.
- Disciplined use of enabling technology is what makes such technology effective.
- Web 2.0 technologies may enable peer-to-peer knowledge transfer in ways that existing enterprisewide knowledge capture applications cannot.
- Engaging the organization in knowledge retention and transfer requires strong change management efforts.
- Using business outcomes to measure the effectiveness of knowledge retention and transfer activities provides the strongest evidence of value.

A Conversation with Dr. John Halamka, CIO of Harvard Medical School and Beth Israel Deaconess Hospital[*]

Through Dr. Halamka's leadership, Harvard Medical School and Beth Israel Deaconess are well on their way into their knowledge management journeys. At Harvard Medical School in 2001, there were hundreds of disconnected Web sites, no central sign on, and no enterprisewide knowledge management system to satisfy the school's administration, educators, students, and research community. By developing MyCourses, an enterprise portal for the organization, various applications came to life. MyCourses serves as a way to unify the knowledge

---

[*] Interview with John Halamka conducted by Jay Liebowitz, June 27, 2008, at Harvard Medical School.

of the people there, and has many features that the users enjoy. Among these are: an automated faculty-activity report generator which, with the push of a button, pulls faculty-article citations from the National Library of Medicine PubMed articles, generates an NIH Biosketch, and automatically formats a CV; an automated feature for department chairs to generate annual reports; 1600 online courses and 200 Flash simulations; problem-based learning using interactive simulations; learning portfolios in a wiki-like fashion; and the hosting of about 300 Harvard Med wikis. The next version of this portal to be launched is called CONNECTS/Catalyst, which will include hyperbolic mapping for linking people at Harvard University with similar research and teaching interests; creating Knowledge Navigators for a kind of Facebook and eBay combination; and incorporating a data-mining algorithm called SHRINE to look for hidden patterns and relationships across the various Harvard databases. Looking toward the immediate future for Harvard Med, there will be an increased focus on social networking, wikis, eBays for knowledge and skills, and finding ways to protect against "skill drain" and "brain drain."

At Beth Israel Deaconess, the board and executive leadership have been very vocal about incorporating knowledge management functions within the daily working lives of their medical community. For example, as of July 1, 2008, all clinicians at Beth Israel Deaconess must be documenting, e-prescribing, and using wikis for lessons learned and problem solving. Every Wednesday from 12 to 2 p.m., the Change Control Board meets to discuss after-action reviews—how did things go this past week, what can we learn, and what change processes and procedures need to be put in place to ensure continued patient safety. This has worked so well that a Change Control Board now also meets at Harvard Medical School to discuss lessons learned and appropriate change processes needed. At Beth Israel Deaconess, the board has mandated that the hospital should eliminate all preventable harm by 2012. To make this happen, knowledge management is playing a key role. Knowledge is being encoded as decision-support rules for patient safety, professional knowledge managers are being used to keep the decision-support rules up to date in the eleven governance-committee areas, wikis and blogs are actively being used, and knowledge is being codified as workflows. Some of the knowledge management work is being outsourced, especially in the decision-support rule development area. Knowledge management's value is being tied to patient safety, return on investment, strategic alignment, or compliance.

Certainly, Harvard Medical School and Beth Israel Deaconess are well into their knowledge management journeys under the leadership of their CIO, Dr. John Halamka, and the support of the boards and executive leadership. They are knowledge management Level 5-type organizations, whereby knowledge management is embedded within the organization and impact is being derived.

The Knowledge Audit

Before developing a knowledge management strategy, an organization should first conduct a knowledge audit to assess the intellectual capital assets of the organization. Similar to a manufacturer taking a physical inventory of its goods, organizations should perform knowledge audits to better understand the nature of their intangible assets. The knowledge audit usually is a Web-based survey, with follow-up interviews, to determine the knowledge use and sharing practices of the employees. Box 1 shows the knowledge audit survey typically used by the author.

Based on the author's experience, the knowledge audit generally takes about three to four months for 500 employees, including the survey customization, survey pilot and fielding, survey completion, survey analysis, and follow-up interviews. The advantages of the knowledge audit are: (1) it provides a better lens through which to view the organization in terms of knowledge management-related practices; (2) it helps identify key types of critical knowledge necessary to the continued growth of the organization; (3) it identifies key individuals who may possess the knowledge; and (4) it provides the foundation for building a knowledge management strategy dealing with people, process, and technology components.

Social Network Analysis

As part of, or separate from, a knowledge audit, some organizations will conduct a social network analysis (SNA) to map knowledge flows and knowledge gaps in the organization. The SNA also will identify people serving in various brokering roles as central connectors, boundary spanners, and peripheral specialists. The central connector is someone who many people go to for certain types of knowledge. The boundary spanner is the liaison between two different groups or departments. The peripheral specialist is the "isolate" who typically works alone and hasn't built a strong network yet.

To stimulate innovation, people need to reach out beyond their own area (Liebowitz, 2007). According to Judith Lamont's article, "Social Networking: KM and Beyond," social networking "has a remarkable ability to involve individuals, often in ways that are unpredictable" (Lamont, 2008). In the May 2008 issue of IEEE Intelligent Systems, Hoffman et al. indicate that finding the knowledge is a challenge for knowledge management researchers and practitioners (Hoffman et al., 2008). This is a true need; as a case in point, Harvard received a $117.5 million Clinical and Translational Science Award on May 29, 2008, to use their CONNECTS/Catalyst portal (as we previously discussed) as a social networking application for seamlessly linking together all the Harvard hospitals and research community (HarvardScience, 2008). The "informal organization" still is poorly understood among most entities. A 2007 report from Katzenbach Partners offers five signs for checking whether your informal organization is alive and well: The word gets out fast; change isn't a dirty word; collaboration is the default mode; employees are tapped in; and stories demonstrate values (Katzenbach Partners, 2007).

The June 3, 2008, cover story in the business section of the *Washington Post* discusses the emerging interest in making all Web sites contain a social networking component. The point is that people like to interact, and applying technology-based approaches to enable this interaction to take place is the future of our professional and personal lives. From scholarly journals such as the *Journal of Knowledge Management* and *Knowledge Management Research and Practice Journal*, to the more popular press such as *Harvard Business Review* and *Newsweek*, all have featured papers dealing with the emergence of social and organizational networking. The success of such initiatives is demonstrated, for example, by the young Facebook social networking site, used by most college and high school students and increasingly more adults, and valued at about $15 billion. Indeed, "one of the most visible trends on the Web is the emergence of social Web sites" (Bojars et al. 2008).

Social networking research highlights the importance of carefully constructing organizations to best leverage knowledge internally and externally. Instead of having "walled gardens," organizations should aim to provide enabling mechanisms to stimulate knowledge discovery, building pathways between these gardens to let "1,000 flowers bloom." To help perform the analysis and visualization of the social networks, SNA tools exist to aid in this process. Two popular tools are: UCINET/ Netdraw (http://www.analytictech.com), a public domain tool; and NetMiner (http://www.netminer.com). There even is the International Network for Social Network Analysis (http://www.insna.org) for additional information about SNA tools, articles, and conferences.

Summary

Knowledge management should be part of an organization's fabric in order to promote innovation, strengthen community, build the institutional memory, and improve "knowledge organization." In the public health sector, knowledge management is a must, since much of the work deals with identifying, sharing, disseminating, and

Box 1: Knowledge Access and Sharing Survey*

A key part of developing a knowledge management strategy is to find out how people gain access to and share knowledge throughout the organization. This survey seeks to gather fairly detailed information about the ways in which you access, share, and use knowledge resources in your work. In answering the questions below, please keep in mind the following: answer for yourself, not how you think someone else in your job might answer; answer for how you actually work now, not how you wish you worked or think you should work.

We expect that some questions will require you to think carefully about the nature of the tasks you perform and how you interact with people both inside and outside the organization day to day. Carefully completing this survey will probably take about 25 minutes. We appreciate your effort in helping us meet a strategic goal designed to make the organization more effective and to make it easier for all of us to do our jobs on a daily basis.

Please forward your completed survey to _____ via e-mail _____ by _____. Thank you!

Please provide the following information:

Name: _____

Which department are you a part of? _____

How long have you been a full-time employee in the organization?
- ☐ Less than 6 months
- ☐ 6 months – less than 1 year
- ☐ 1 year – less than 3 years
- ☐ 3 years – less than 5 years
- ☐ More than 5 years

In the course of doing your job, which resource do you most often turn to first when looking for information? (please, check only one)
- ☐ E-mail or talk to a colleague in the organization
- ☐ E-mail or talk to a colleague who works outside the organization
- ☐ Do a global Web search (for example, Google, Yahoo!)
- ☐ Go to a known Web site
- ☐ Search online organization resources (for example, intranet)
- ☐ Search through documents/publications in your office
- ☐ Post a message on a Listserv/online community to which you belong
- ☐ Ask your manager for guidance based on his/her experience
- ☐ Other (*please specify*) _____

---

* Developed by Dr. Jay Liebowitz, JHU, jliebow1@jhu.edu.

BOX 1 Continued

What would be your second course of action from the above list? _____

_____

Think about the times when you've been really frustrated by not having a critical piece of knowledge or information you needed to get something done at the organization. Give an example, including the nature of the challenge and how the need eventually was met.

_____
_____
_____

Knowledge Resources

How often *on average* do you use each of the following to do your job?

	Daily	*Weekly*	*Monthly*	*Quarterly*	*Never*
Organization-wide database	☐	☐	☐	☐	☐
Organization-operated Web site (e.g., intranet)	☐	☐	☐	☐	☐
Department- or division-operated database (e.g., shared calendar)	☐	☐	☐	☐	☐
My own database or contact list file	☐	☐	☐	☐	☐
Organization policy/ procedures manual or guidelines	☐	☐	☐	☐	☐
Department- or division-specific procedures manual or guidelines	☐	☐	☐	☐	☐
Vendor-provided procedures manual or guidelines	☐	☐	☐	☐	☐
My own notes or procedures	☐	☐	☐	☐	☐

List up to five resources (hard copy or Web-based) that you use to perform your job, and indicate how often you use them. These resources can be journals, magazines, newsletters, books, Web sites, and so forth.

	Daily	*Weekly*	*Monthly*	*Quarterly*
1.	☐	☐	☐	☐
2.	☐	☐	☐	☐
3.	☐	☐	☐	☐
4.	☐	☐	☐	☐
5.	☐	☐	☐	☐

How often *on average* do you ask each of the following staff for help with understanding or clarifying how you are to perform your job, solving a problem, getting an answer to a question from a customer, or learning how to accomplish a new task?

	Daily	*Weekly*	*Monthly*	*Quarterly*	*Never*
Your immediate supervisor	☐	☐	☐	☐	☐
Your department head	☐	☐	☐	☐	☐
Your division head	☐	☐	☐	☐	☐
Subject-matter expert (in an area of policy, practice, or research)	☐	☐	☐	☐	☐
Technical or functional expert (e.g., accounting, legal, contracts administration, technology)	☐	☐	☐	☐	☐
A peer or colleague in your department or division (informal)	☐	☐	☐	☐	☐
A peer or colleague outside your department or division (informal)	☐	☐	☐	☐	☐

(continued)

BOX 1 Continued

Name the top three people, in order, to whom you go when you have questions or seek advice in the following areas:

	One	*Two*	*Three*
General advice			
Management and leadership knowledge/advice			
Subject-matter expertise/content knowledge			
Institutional/historical knowledge about the foundation			
Technical/procedural knowledge			

List up to five experts *outside* the organization whom you access to do your job. For each one, please indicate *on average* how often you contact them.

	Daily	*Weekly*	*Monthly*	*Quarterly*
1.	☐	☐	☐	☐
2.	☐	☐	☐	☐
3.	☐	☐	☐	☐
4.	☐	☐	☐	☐
5.	☐	☐	☐	☐

Knowledge Use

Which of the following do you *usually* use and/or perform (that is, on a daily or weekly basis) in doing your job? (*check all that apply*)

☐ Data or information from a known source (e.g., database, files) you have to retrieve to answer a specific question.

☐ Data or information you have to gather yourself from multiple sources and analyze and/or synthesize to answer a specific question.

☐ Instruction (step by step) you provide (that is, not a document) to a customer, vendor, or staff person.

☐ Direction you provide to a customer, vendor, or staff person (such as advice, counsel, or guidance, not step by step).

☐ Judgments or recommendations you are asked to make based on data or information that is given to you.

☐ Judgments or recommendations you are asked to make based on data or information that you must find yourself.

☐ Routine procedure or process for handling information, paperwork, requests, payments, invoices, and so forth (always done the same way).

☐ Variable procedure or process for handling information, paperwork, requests, payments, invoices, and so forth (requires some analysis and judgment to select the proper procedure or process to follow).

☐ Reports, memoranda, letters, or informational materials for customers, vendors, or staff that you must compile and/or write.

☐ Educational or promotional materials that you must compile and/or write.

☐ Proposals you develop to recommend new programs, projects, procedures, or processes.

After you have received, gathered, or produced information, instructions, documents, proposals, etc., what do you do with them after you have completed the task? (*check all that apply*)

☐ Save them in an electronic file in my personal directory.
☐ Save them in an electronic file in a shared directory (e.g., p:drive, intranet).
☐ Save them in a personal paper file.
☐ Save them in a secure departmental paper file.
☐ Save them in an open departmental paper file.
☐ Share them or distribute them to others.
☐ Delete or toss them.
☐ Other (*please specify*) _____ ■

Sharing

When you come across a news item, article, magazine, book, Web site, announcement for a meeting or course, or some other information that may be useful to other organization staff, what are you *most likely* to do? (*check only one*)

☐ Tell them about it or distribute a copy to them personally.
☐ Post an announcement on the intranet.

(continued)

BOX 1 Continued

☐ Send a broadcast e-mail.
☐ Send a memo or a copy through the interoffice mail.
☐ Intend to share it but usually too busy to follow through.
☐ Include it in the weekly update.
☐ Ignore it.
☐ Other (*please specify*) _____

What are the constraints you face in being able to access or share knowledge?

_____

_____

What critical knowledge is at risk of being lost in your department or division because of turnover and lack of backup expertise?

_____

_____

Training/Tools

When you want to learn or improve a skill or task, what do you prefer to do? (*check all that apply*)

☐ Get formal face-to-face training or course work outside the work place.
☐ Get formal, self-directed training (e.g., workbook, CD-ROM, online course).
☐ Have a specialist train me onsite.
☐ Train myself (informally, using a manual or tutorial program).
☐ Have my supervisor show me how to do it.
☐ Have a friend or colleague show me how to do it.
☐ Other (*please specify*) _____

What kind of tools or resources do you prefer to help you do your job? (*check all that apply*)

☐ Person I can talk to in real time.
☐ Help line or help desk via phone, fax, or e-mail.
☐ Advice via online communities of practice (on the intranet, Listservs, or other sources).
☐ Printed documents (e.g., resource books, manuals).
☐ Electronic documents.
☐ Audiovisual/multimedia material.
☐ Special software.
☐ Web-based utility, directory, or service.
☐ Other (*please specify*) _____

Knowledge Needs

What information or knowledge that you do not currently have would you like to have to do your job better? Consider all aspects of your job, including administrative tasks, policies and procedures, interpersonal relationships, and so forth.

_____

_____

_____

_____

What information or knowledge that the organization currently does not have do you think it should or will need to have to execute its mission, improve organizational effectiveness, and serve its customers with excellence? (You may answer for specific departments as well as for the organization as a whole.)

_____

_____

_____

_____

To what extent do you agree with the following statements:

	Strongly disagree	Disagree	No opinion	Agree	Strongly agree
I would benefit from having access to documents that contain introductory knowledge that I currently have to acquire from experts directly.	☐	☐	☐	☐	☐
I would benefit from templates to help me more easily capture knowledge (e.g., standard format for documenting what I learned at a conference or meeting).	☐	☐	☐	☐	☐

(continued)

BOX 1 Continued

	Strongly disagree	Disagree	No opinion	Agree	Strongly agree
I would benefit from processes to help me contribute knowledge that I don't currently document or share.	☐	☐	☐	☐	☐
I would benefit from support to determine the most relevant knowledge to share for various audiences and how best to share it.	☐	☐	☐	☐	☐
I have knowledge in areas that I know the organization could benefit from but no way to make it available.	☐	☐	☐	☐	☐

Knowledge Flow

Imagine that you've just won your organization's first Knowledge Sharing Award. This award is given to a person who shares his or her mission- or operation-critical knowledge so that the organization can be more effective. List the top five categories of knowledge that earned you this award and the category of staff with whom you shared it.

	Knowledge Category	Staff Category
1.		
2.		
3.		
4.		
5.		

How can the knowledge flow in your area of responsibility be improved?

_____

_____

_____

_____

Additional Comments

_____

_____

_____

_____

_____

Thank you for taking the time to complete this survey.

creating knowledge. In the next chapter, we will take a look at examples where knowledge management is being used in public health. Thereafter, specific case studies of knowledge management in action in the public health arena will be presented.

References

Bojars, U., et al. 2008. Interlinking the social Web with semantics. IEEE Intelligent Systems. 23(3):29.

HarvardScience newsletter. May 2008. http://harvardscience.harvard.edu.

Hoffman, R., et al. 2008. Knowledge management revisited. IEEE Intelligent Systems, 23(3)84–8.

Lamont, J. 2008. Social networking: KM and beyond. *KMWorld* 17(6):13–14.

Liebowitz, J. 2007. *Social Networking: The Essence of Innovation*, Lanham, Md.: Scarecrow Press.

Katzenbach Partners. 2007. The informal organization. Available at http://www.katzenback .com.

Chapter 2

Knowledge Management and Public Health

A Winning Combination

Jay Liebowitz, Richard A. Schieber,
and Joanne D. Andreadis

Contents

Introduction

A literature review of knowledge management and public health reveals growing
interest in applying knowledge management principles, methods, and applications

in the public health arena. Key reasons for this interest include the following (Association of State and Territorial Health Officials, 2005a): capturing knowledge to ensure public health preparedness, managing information more effectively, enabling public health professionals to work collaboratively in a virtual environment, and improving effectiveness in the face of dwindling resources. Revere et al. (2007) iterate that comprehensive, coordinated, and accessible information is needed to meet the demands of the public health workforce. The Association of State and Territorial Health Officials (2005a, 2005b) highlights the key functions where knowledge management can aid public health officials:

Monitor: health status to identify and solve community health problems.
Diagnose and investigate: health problems and health hazards in the community.
Inform, educate, and empower: people about health issues.
Mobilize: community partnerships to identify and solve health problems.
Develop: policies and plans that support individual and community health efforts.
Enforce: laws and regulations that protect health and ensure safety.
Link: people to needed personal health services and assure the provision of health care.
Assure: a competent public and personal health care workforce.
Evaluate: effectiveness, accessibility, and quality of personal and population-based health services.
Research: new insights and innovative solutions to health problems.

Knowledge management for health appeared on the radar screen of health-care stakeholders about five to eight years ago (Dwivedi et al., 2005). Although knowledge exists in all health care organizations, it often remains in silos or on the sidelines, not used to its maximum potential or to achieve strategic results (Macdonald, 2003). In 1991, Dr. Donald Berwick, identified the need to transfer quality improvement practices developed outside the health care industry to reduce cost and manage continual improvement of products, services, and services within health care. Acknowledging the need to develop a knowledge management process, he founded the Institute for Healthcare Improvement, which was chartered to "develop, test, and implement a system for accelerating improvement by spreading ideas within and between organizations" as a conduit to rapidly bridge the gap between best practice and common practice (Massoud et al., 2006). Both knowledge management and clinical governance need to share the same criteria to operate (Plaice and Kitch, 2003). Advanced knowledge management for community health should expedite the transfer of research evidence to practice and provide essential logistical support for action (Balas and Krishna, 2004). Knowledge management will be a major responsibility of health care management (Gray, 2008). Knowledge management research in influential journals always has had well-articulated theoretical perspectives, research paradigms, and research methods (Guo and Sheffield, 2008). Findings indicate that health care providers must better cooperate and communicate with one another (Sanchez and Cegarra, 2008).

Knowledge management is being applied to public health and health care in a number of ways (Guptill, 2005): communities of practice, content management, knowledge and capability transfer, performance results tracking, and technology and support infrastructure. Several examples of knowledge management efforts in the public health field are listed in Table 2.1. The World Health Organization's knowledge management strategy (http://www.who.int/kms/en) focuses on strengthening country health systems through better knowledge management, establishing knowledge management in public health, and enabling WHO to become a better learning organization by improving access to the world's health information, translating knowledge into policy and action, sharing and reapplying experiential knowledge, leveraging e-health in countries, and fostering an enabling environment. WHO is promoting knowledge implementation for bridging the "do–know" gap (the routine application of established evidence-based practices). Another example is TEPHINET, a nonprofit, global public health network that links field-based epidemiology training programs, such as the Epidemic Intelligence Service of the U.S. Centers for Disease Control and Prevention's Field Epidemiology Training Programs, The Rockefeller Foundation's Public Health Schools without Walls, and the European Programme for Intervention Epidemiology Training to share knowledge and best practices to rapidly strengthen global public health capacity. Other knowledge management work in public health supports an online registry of reviews evaluating the effectiveness of public health and health promotion interventions (Dobbins et al., 2004). This registry is one component of a comprehensive national public health knowledge transfer strategy. Communities of practice are being actively used in the public health and health care fields, such as the community of practice with intensive care units for exchange of information and knowledge (Rolls et al., 2008). According to Fahey et al. (2003), the knowledge network is more likely to be successful if its priorities are maximizing scarce resources, identification of expertise, education, and knowledge management. An earlier study by Atkinson and Gold (2001) resulted in consensus on thirty-four functions and thirty-two output/content elements of a proposed Web-based knowledge management system in health care called PreventionEffects.net. Later chapters in the book will highlight some of the key knowledge management work being pursued in public health by leading organizations worldwide.

As with any emerging field, knowledge management presents challenges to public health officials. Some of these challenges include (Association of State and Territorial Health Officials, 2005a): lack of leadership commitment; lack of understanding of an organization's business processes, cultural barriers, lack of processes for data sharing and reuse, scope of content, and lack of appropriate technology and skills. Additional barriers to information access are time, resource reliability, trustworthiness and credibility of information, and information overload (Plaice and Kitch, 2003). Others have indicated the challenges of knowledge management

Table 2.1   Examples of Knowledge Management Efforts in Public Health

Listserv and community of practice	NSW Intensive Care Coordination and Monitoring Unit, Australia
Managed-knowledge networks	NHS Scotland
MedGrid—an integrative healthcare knowledge service mechanism	China
UK public health network	U.K.
Embedding knowledge management in the National Health Service	U.K.
Dutch knowledge infrastructure program for occupational health professionals	The Netherlands
Developing a comprehensive national public health knowledge transfer strategy	McMaster University, Canada
Knowledge exchange	Canadian Health Services Research Foundation
Virtual network for community health research	Alberta Heritage Foundation for Medical Research, Canada
Knowledge systems in health; after-action reviews	WHO (World Health Organization)
Knowledge translation in global health	WHO
Social networking	The World Bank, WHO, PAHO (Pan American Health Organization)
Knowledge management for global nutrition	USAID (United States Agency for International Development)
National Health Knowledge Infrastructure	National Health Information Infrastructure initiative
Knowledge, information, and data sharing	NIH/NLM (National Institutes of Health/National Library of Medicine)
Portal aimed at public health professionals	CDC
PulseNet/PulseNet International for data and knowledge sharing to assist outbreak response	CDC

CDC GlobalHealth.net	CDC
PEPFAR.net	CDC
Model Practice Database and quarterly NACCHO Exchange: Model Practices	National Association of County and City Health Officials
myPublicHealth	University of Washington
Knowledge transfer	JHPIEGO (Johns Hopkins)
PreventionEffects.net	University of Maryland
Medical data mining	Stanford University
Communities of practice	Public Health Informatics Institute
Cataloging knowledge	California Department of Health Services
Web-based knowledge management dashboard	Kentucky Department of Public Health

as volume of information, information security, quality, and the ability to access and use information (Association of State and Territorial Health Officials, 2005b). According to Pablos and Shademani (2006), organizations lack a fostering environment—including incentives and rewards systems—to encourage and enhance sharing, learning, and applying and reapplying knowledge for problem solving. King and Marks' work (2008) unexpectedly suggests the impact of local supervisory control (economic agency theory motivators) has more of an influence on both the frequency and quality of knowledge sharing than organizational support motivators.

Drivers for Change

As we consider how public health will evolve to better address new challenges, we see several key driving forces that support broader adoption of knowledge management: the globalization of public health, resource constraints, changing needs and expectations of people, and technological advancement.

Globalization of Public Health

The global eradication of smallpox is the best public health triumph of the past century (World Health Organization, 2000). Its eradication exemplifies the importance of knowledge management, as the success of the program required both a coordinated global public health campaign that focused on mass vaccination, and the development of surveillance systems to find cases and outbreaks to support focused containment measures (Centers for Disease Control and Prevention, 2007). Efficient knowledge management that crosses organizational, community, cultural, national, and geographical boundaries is essential to ensure that the right information reaches the right destination as quickly as possible. In 2006, Larry Brilliant, M.D., M.P.H., identified "early detection and early response" as the key factors that led to the first successful eradication of any disease. Many lessons can be learned from both the successes and failures encountered during the eradication of smallpox, but the world around us has changed, and what succeeded in the past may not be sufficient to meet future public health needs. The increasing interconnectedness of the world now allows more rapid and widespread transmission of disease and dissemination of unhealthy behaviors or practices, and necessitates the development of effective knowledge management systems that support early detection and response to public health threats.

In *The World is Flat: A Brief History of the Twenty-first Century*, Tom Friedman identified ten flatteners that leveled the competitive playing fields between industrial and emerging markets throughout the world (2005). The flattening of the global economy and technological advances of the last fifty years have accelerated the globalization of health and in the process created new opportunities and threats for public health (Yach and Bettcher, 1998). Infectious disease always has had the potential to cause pandemics, but because of the globalization of economies, transportation systems, communication, and food supplies, among other influen-cers, the threat of a pandemic may be greater and now extends to other areas of public health, such as chronic disease. Thus, the interconnectedness between disparate geographical locations or societies is leading to health events far away increasingly having a local impact, and vice versa (Fidler, 2001). Examples that demonstrate the flattening global health landscape include the SARS global outbreak of 2003, which spread from Guandong province in China to rapidly infect more than 8,000 people in thirty-seven countries around the world; the spread of HIV; the potential pandemic threat of avian influenza A (H5N1); and international food safety events. Additional examples include the health outcomes of transboundary environmental pollution, tobacco commerce, and standards of occupational health and safety. The flattening of global public health also means we must grapple with and solve more than one public health problem at a time and focus on the interactions and connections among health-related problems. The Syndemics Prevention Network offers a means to assemble information that provides a systems view of public health involving two or more afflictions that synergistically contribute to the burden of disease in a population (Milstein, 2008). Having knowledge management capacity to create the connections between clusters of health-related issues is critical to establishing interventions and policies that account for the relationship and aggregate impact of public health challenges, such as substance abuse, violence, and AIDS.

Our increasingly difficult, widespread, and interconnected public health challenges require us to collect timely, comprehensive information from diverse sources and to convert that information into knowledge that supports actions or policies with tangible health impact. To better address global public health challenges, we must share information more efficiently and implement policies, practices, and methods that can effectively bridge the "know–do" gap. The flattening global health landscape clearly will promote networked cross-sector collaboration and accelerate the general adoption of knowledge management practices in public health.

Resource Constraints

In addition to facing daunting global public health challenges that require complex problem solving, many organizations are affected by the global economic crisis. The central paradox is that public health resources (human capital and financial) are being reduced at a time when demand for such services most certainly will increase. A 2008 survey of 1,079 local health departments in the United State that was conducted by the National Association of County and City Health Officials (NACCHO) found that more than half of local health departments laid off employees or are unable to replace employees lost from attrition caused by budget restrictions (NACCHO, 2009). Extrapolating the results of the respondents from that survey to all 2,422 local public health departments suggest between 3,000 and 6,000 local public health workers lost their jobs in 2008, and more are expected to lose their jobs in 2009 because of budget limitations. Additionally, an Association of Schools of Public Health (ASPH, 2008) report indicates that the current local, state, and federal workforce is inadequate to meet U.S. and global public health needs. Using the 1980 ratio of 220 public health workers to U.S. population as a benchmark, the ASPH report projects the need for an additional 250,000 public health workers (or total of 738,771) by 2020 to avert a workforce shortage and public health crisis (ASPH, 2008; Helsing and Anderson, 2008). On the global stage, some of the greatest deficits in the public health workforce occur in developing regions, such as sub-Saharan Africa, which represents 11 percent of the world's population and 24 percent of the global disease burden (World Health Report, 2006), including 67 percent of all people living with HIV and 75 percent of all AIDS deaths in 2007 (UNAIDS, 2008). In addition to the attrition from economic loss, as well as from other reasons, the graying of the public health workforce also causes considerable concern. ASPH estimates suggest that more than 40 percent of the current federal public health workforce is eligible to retire and that by 2012 more than 23 percent of the federal, state, and local public health workforce (>110,000 workers) will retire (ASPH, 2008). In short, public health will once again be called to do more with less, while enduring unprecedented loss of critical expertise.

Although knowledge management cannot replace lost public health workers, it can enable an organization to retain critical knowledge and informal knowledge networks. As in any field, public health solutions are based on information, both explicit (written, spoken, or known, or a combination of these) and tacit (undocumented but available by asking). One role of knowledge management is to capture and use tacit and explicit information to improve information flow and develop new information that will directly benefit public health. For example, one of the functions of knowledge management is to improve institutional memory by developing a system that documents how and why things are done. Capturing institutional memory is particularly important for the federal government and other organizations facing a graying workforce or high attrition. Furthermore, institutionalization of knowledge is very important in the context of unstable staffing. Considering the current economic crisis, with sudden and unexpected reductions already occurring in the public health workforce, knowledge management becomes a critical mechanism to ensure quality performance and the continuity of public health's ability to protect health and promote health equity.

Changing Needs and Expectations of People

The changing needs and expectations of the public we serve also drive the need to broadly adopt knowledge management practices in public health. For example, the number of individuals aged 65 years and older is expected to double in the next 30 years from today's 37 million people (Federal Interagency Forum on Aging-Related Statistics, 2008). Advances in infectious disease control (such as sanitation, vaccination, and antibiotics) have created substantial global gains in the life expectancy of infants and children. Technological advances in medicine also have lowered mortality later in life. As a result, within two decades the number of people over 60 years old is expected to exceed those who are less than 24 years of age (Bloom and Canning, 2005). Thus, although infectious disease control was a principal driver in the beginning of the last century, noncommunicable disease and disability resulting from heart disease, diabetes, and other chronic diseases—which in large part are preventable and are outcomes of behavior and lifestyle factors—will become an increasing focus for public health and health care (Lee, 2007). This important paradigm shift means that as more people survive into late adulthood, the public health impact of lifestyle factors, such as diet, the built environment, inactivity, and air quality, will become more evident. This increased impact from lifestyle factors will require public health to collect information from a variety of sources and subsequently identify both obvious and hidden linkages that adversely impact health. Consequently, public health experts will need to accelerate the process of establishing an evidence base and then translating that knowledge into practices that create informed policy and promote more healthful behaviors.

Another interesting facet of public expectation is the high level of technological savvy exhibited across the population—beginning with the millennial generation (born between 1980 and 2000) through to aging baby boomers (born between 1946 and 1964). This technological savvy translates to into an empowered, mobile public that has access to an immense amount of information. Thus, a growing proportion of the general population is open to receiving and transmitting personal and nonpersonal information in a wide array of new platforms (such as personal health records, social network smoking-cessation programs, genome databases, and self-reporting Web sites, such as "Patients Like Me"). Furthermore, this empowered public will be more proactively and directly engaged in public health issues than ever before. Technologies will empower the public by linking behavior, lifestyle factors, and their local environment to their personal health and by supporting the cooperative action and advocacy of self-assembled groups around communal issues. These changes in perspective present new opportunities and challenges for public health by altering how people and public health organizations interact and changing the way in which information is collected, developed into knowledge, and disseminated.

Technological Advancement

Technology is an undisputed enabler of knowledge management. Mainstream adoption of the Internet, development of sensor-aware environments, high-capacity computing, and social communication platforms have made information a commodity and forever altered how it is collected, accessed, transmitted, disseminated, and networked. As an enabler, technology does not replace human interaction but rather overcomes barriers of time, space, and scale. In the late 1700s, it may have taken months or years for most of the public to learn the outcome of U.S. presidential elections; now almost everyone knows the outcome of an election almost as soon as voting ends. Although technology is not a panacea for establishing organizational knowledge management, it is essential for creating, sharing, and storing knowledge. For example, the conversion between tacit and explicit knowledge—which is critical for optimal organizational performance and creation of new knowledge—is greatly facilitated through wikis, e-mail, Web-based video, chat rooms, forums, and Web-based social networks. IBM uses a global, Web-based forum called the IBM InnovationJam that enables thousands of employees and guests from around the world to exchange ideas, capture information, and share experiential knowledge on strategic topics of interest. Intellipedia is a wiki-based online system created by the intelligence community to broadly share information and engage a more youthful workforce (Shrader, 2006). A recent report demonstrates that Intellipedia contains more than 35,000 articles and has more than 37,000 users (Havenstein, 2008). Technology is thus also well suited to facilitate rapid identification of information or individuals with specific knowledge in a given area. Future advances in artificial intelligence will help to better "sense" information and link individuals to the most relevant material, people, or places to improve the speed and the flow of useful knowledge. This improved speed and flow is critical in equipping people (within and outside of public health) to most effectively use the deluge of information available at any given time. Technology also is spurring the creation of a global health commons—engaging traditional and nontraditional public health partners to promote health as a sustainable, collectively maintained resource. Specifically, Web 2.0 has spawned new tools that can be adapted to support the key public health functions identified in the beginning of this chapter.

For example, ICARE (http://icare/ieor/berkeley.edu) is a social network that helps communities provide efficient, grassroots solutions to disaster relief by enabling peer-to-peer matching of individual donors and recipients of aid. Patientslikeme (http://www.patientslikeme.com) allows patients to capture and share information, ideas, and experiences with each other, health professionals, and professional organizations. "Who Is Sick?" (http://whoissick.org), allows individuals to use geomapping tools to report symptoms and create real-time lay epidemiology profiles. These examples highlight the potential for Web or mobile networks to support key public health functions by dramatically amplifying the flow of information through vast networks of people. Public and nonprofit organizations already have started using wikis, blogs, microblogging, tags, Really Simple Syndication (RSS), and other Web 2.0 tools as knowledge collection and distribution tools. As an example, the Red Cross, Office of National Drug Control Policy, and Centers for Disease Control and Prevention have already embraced microblogging tools such as Twitter. Others, such as the U.S. Geological Survey, operate sites such as "Did You Feel It?" that allow citizens to report earthquake activity. The use of social media (such as Flickr, Twitter, Wikipedia, YouTube, and Google Maps) in grassroots emergency response also has been demonstrated in the United States during the Virginia Tech campus shootings and California wildfires to convey real-time local knowledge (Palmer, 2009). Certainly, there are questions concerning the present accuracy and quality of information that need to be addressed, but the potential for Web 2.0 to support public health knowledge management is tremendous.

A discussion of the impact of technology on public health knowledge management would be incomplete without mentioning cell phones and other mobile devices (commonly equipped with GPS, video, camera, and text messaging). The availability of wireless networks has enabled poor countries with minimal public health infrastructure to leapfrog older technologies and use cell phones to establish health information architectures and surveillance programs, and to provide remote medical treatment or diagnosis. In Kenya, mobile device applications enable health officials to collect information on specific patients, symptoms, treatments, and medical supplies/vaccines and to obtain instantaneous feedback during public health outbreaks (United Nations Foundation, 2007). Similarly, the public-private partnership "Phones for Health" program has helped countries such as Rwanda develop a national-scale, real-time public health information system that assists health workers to manage HIV/AIDS services and exchange treatment guidelines (United States President's Emergency Plan for AIDS Relief, 2007). Of course, the utility of mobile health platforms is not unique to developing nations, and this technology has great potential for integrating public health into daily living by promoting healthy behavior and enhancing communication between individuals and their health providers. This powerful combination of technology with an empowered, proactive public will foster the creation of new knowledge and innovation—a winning combination for public health.

Adoption of Knowledge Management: Practical Steps

If the adoption of knowledge management by public health departments is a current priority, then how should it begin? The structure of potentially developing knowledge management in an organization can be envisioned with the basic functions positioned on the bottom row of the pyramid (Figure 2.1):

- Adopting a senior champion in the organization to support knowledge management efforts and develop a working group
- Educating the staff on knowledge management
- Determining how and where knowledge management might be of particular benefit to the organization
- Determining how people in the organization are connected through social networks
- Developing knowledge management initiatives (e.g., best-practice directory, lessons-learned database, communities of practice, expertise locators, collaborative systems, and e-learning systems)
- Tracking individual efforts in knowledge management as part of the annual personnel appraisal
- Developing leading and lagging measurements (that include inputs, outputs, and outcomes) to track and evaluate progress

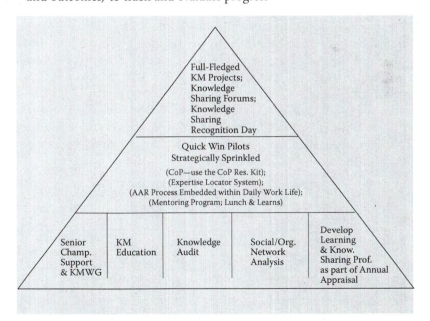

Figure 2.1   Building blocks for a KM program.

Those leading the knowledge management effort of the organization will want to become informed users and advisers of knowledge management principles and methods. Fortunately, that task is relatively simple thanks to the Internet (the largest and most well used of all knowledge management projects). A few Web sites have more than enough information for those leading the development of knowledge management to get started (Table 2.2). Organizations developed to promote knowledge management, such as the Knowledge Management Professional Society, provide support using blogs, discussion forums, Listserv, and downloadable information. Journals such the *Journal of Knowledge Management, Knowledge Management Research and Practice Journal, International Journal of Knowledge Management, Expert Systems with Applications Journal,* and others are a source for review articles and up-to-date information.

A critical factor in establishing a knowledge management program is creating a foundation built on transparency and trust coupled with accountability and reward. High-impact, less-difficult projects are creating communities of practice, wikis, and blogs; developing mentoring to support knowledge management and holding brown-bag seminars; storytelling; and job shadowing and job rotation (Figure 2.2). Note that some of these functions already exist in many organizations. For example, storytelling can be used as a mechanism to convey difficult-to-uncover tacit knowledge in a manner that is easily understood. One way to apply storytelling in a professional environment is to use part of a staff meeting to describe what worked and what did not work as a project progresses. Another basic function is analyzing formal and informal organizational social networks to identify how knowledge flows and where there are gaps in knowledge. Another function is to identify key players with specific roles in the organization, such as central connectors, boundary spanners, and those who are relatively isolated from others in the system. In nearly all organizations, e-mail is a key means of rapidly communicating information one on one or one on many. Listservs are commonly used to gather information from all members and in turn pass it quickly to all members for comment. Word-processing applications and wikis track changes and comments made to work products by each author or reviewer. The Semantic Web and Web 2.0 will enhance the capability of

Table 2.2 Useful Knowledge Management-Related Web Sites

• Http://www.km.gov (Federal KM Working Group)
• Http://kmpro.org (KM Professional Society)
• Http://www.insna.org (International Network of Social Network Analysts)
• Http://www.ejkm.com (Electronic Journal of KM)
• Http://www.kmworld.com (KMWorld)
• Http://www.who.int/kms/en (KM at WHO)

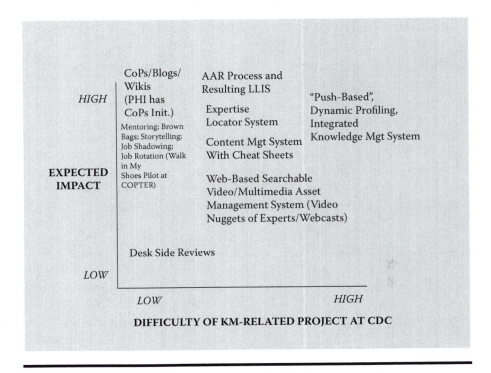

Figure 2.2 KM project impact and level of difficulty.

organizations to grow knowledge management through social networking, as many Web sites have a built-in social networking component.

Components can be added to an organization either one at a time, serially, or in clusters, depending on the existing capacity of the health department and its relative commitment to using knowledge management. Leaders in an organization should avoid the mistake of tackling a high-level function in the knowledge management pyramid before the functions in underlying layers are established within an organization. Attempting to develop those higher functions too early before the processes that support them are in place will increase the likelihood that knowledge management in the organization will fail.

Through basic operations such as these, a knowledge management system can be developed or enhanced to permit information to be accessed and used more easily. Such information can be the source of important "discoveries" through research conducted via knowledge management by research scientists, epidemiologists, statisticians, economists, and social scientists. Advanced knowledge management technologies, such as mining data, text, multimedia, and Web content, can help discover hidden patterns and relationships in large masses of data, text, and images gathered for populations. Such an approach may have value in predicting, diagnosing, and helping respond definitively to acute outbreaks and chronic diseases in the community.

The Future of Knowledge Management in Public Health

Most public health agencies already are concerned with many of the processes involved in knowledge management: identifying and capturing, sharing, applying, and creating knowledge. Locating and using experts and communities for identifying, sharing, and transferring knowledge will be increasingly important for public health applications. Developing ontologies for allowing ease of use and access to knowledge management systems will support broader adoption for public health applications. Advanced technologies, such as data mining, text mining, multimedia mining, and Web mining, also will achieve greater prominence as discovering hidden patterns and relationships in large masses of data, text, and images becomes increasingly essential for connecting the dots in public health-related issues and outbreaks.

Social networking and the application of social network analysis will continue to be applied to identify knowledge flows, knowledge gaps, brokering roles, informal networks, and more formal ones. Certainly, the Semantic Web and Web 2.0 will influence social networking, as many Web sites will have a social networking component built in. Social network analysis will help identify the central connectors, boundary spanners, and isolates as related to public health applications.

In the same way that the cell phone is ubiquitous, knowledge management also will be seamlessly embedded within the fabric of organizations and society. We already have been applying knowledge management concepts for eons, perhaps under different terminology. As knowledge management becomes a part of the daily lives of individuals, people will have increased means for capturing, exchanging, and creating knowledge. Those public health organizations that embrace knowledge management now will have a head start for taking advantage of tomorrow's windows of opportunity.

> **Disclaimer:** The views and opinions of the authors expressed herein do not necessarily state or reflect those of the CDC, HHS, or the United States government.

Bibliography

Association of Schools of Public Health. 2008. Confronting the public health workforce crisis: ASPH statement on the public health workforce. Available at http://www.asph.org/UserFiles/PHWFShortage0208.pdf. Retrieved on Dec. 12, 2008.

Association of State and Territorial Health Officials. 2004. State public health employee worker shortage report, a civil service recruitment and retention crisis. Washington, D.C.

Association of State and Territorial Health Officials. 2005a. Knowledge management for public health professionals. Washington, D.C.

Association of State and Territorial Health Officials. 2005b. Examples of knowledge management in public health practice. Washington, D.C.

Association of State and Territorial Health Officials. 2007. ASTHO state public health survey. Washington, D.C.

Atkinson, N. and R. Gold. 2001. Online research to guide knowledge management planning. *Health Education Research* 16(6).

Balas, E. and S. Krishna. 2004. From SARS to systems: Developing advanced knowledge management for public health. *Studies in Health Technology and Informatics* 100.

Bali, R. and A. Dwivedi, eds. 2007. *Healthcare Knowledge Management: Issues, Advances, and Successes.* Springer.

Becerra, I. and D. Leidner, eds. 2008. *Knowledge Management: An Evolutionary View.* Advances in MIS Series. M.E. Sharpe Publishers, Armonk, NY.

Bloom, D. and D. Canning. 2005. Global demographic change: Dimensions and economic significance. Working Paper 1. Harvard initiative for global health, program on the global demography of aging. Boston.

Brilliant, Larry: TED Prize wish: Help stop the next pandemic. Streaming video 2006. TED conference. Available at http://www.ted.com/talks/view/id/58. Retrieved on Jan. 20, 2009.

Centers for Disease Control and Prevention. 2007. Smallpox: 30th anniversary of global eradication. Available at http://www.cdc.gov/Features/SmallpoxEradication. Retrieved on Jan. 22, 2009.

Dobbins, M., K. DeCorby, and T. Twiddy. 2004. A knowledge transfer strategy for public health decision makers. *Worldviews on Evidence-Based Nursing.*

Dwivedi, A., R. Bali, and R. Naguib. 2005. Implications for healthcare knowledge management systems: A case study, proceedings of the IEEE Engineering in Medicine and Biology Conference.

Fahey, D., E. Carson, D. Cramp, and M. Gray. 2003. User requirements and understanding of public health networks in England. *Journal of Epidemiology and Community Health* 57.

Federal Interagency Forum on Aging-Related Statistics. 2008. Americans living longer, enjoying greater health and prosperity, but important disparities remain, says federal report. Press release. Available at http://www.agingstats.gov/agingstatsdotnet/Main_Site/Data/2008_Documents/Embargoed_PR.pdf. Retrieved Oct. 10, 2008.

Fidler, D.P. 2001. The globalization of public health: The first 100 years of international health diplomacy. *Bulletin of the World Health Organization* 79(9):842–49.

Gray, M. 2008. Making the future of healthcare. *Journal of Z. Evid. Forbild. Qual. Gesunsh. Wesen.* Elsevier.

Guo, Z. and J. Sheffield. 2008. A paradigmatic and methodological examination of knowledge management research: 2000 to 2004. *Decision Support Systems,* 44.

Guptill, J. 2005. Knowledge management in health care. *Journal of Health Care Finance* 31(3).

Havenstein, H. 2008. Top secret: CIA explains its Wikipedia-like national security project. Computerworld. Retrieved Jan. 10, 2009.

Helsing, K. and Anderson, S. Feb. 27, 2008. More than 250,000 additional public health workers needed by 2020 to avert public health crisis. News release. Association of Schools of Public Health. Washington, D.C.

King, W. and P. Marks. 2008. Motivating knowledge sharing through a knowledge management system. *Omega* 36.

Lee, M. 2007. Global health and population aging. Today's Research on Aging. Population Reference Bureau, 4.

Liebowitz, J. 2004. *Addressing the Human Capital Crisis in the Federal Government: A Knowledge Management Perspective.* Boston: Elsevier/Butterworth-Heinemann.

Liebowitz, J. 2006a. *What They Didn't Tell You About Knowledge Management*. Lanham, Md.: Scarecrow Press.

Liebowitz, J., ed. 2006b. *Strategic Intelligence: Business Intelligence, Competitive Intelligence, and Knowledge Management*. New York: Auerbach Publishing/Taylor & Francis.

Liebowitz, J. 2007. *Social Networking: The Essence of Innovation*. Lanham, Md.: Scarecrow Press.

Liebowitz, J., ed. 2008. *Making Cents Out of Knowledge Management*. Lanham, Md.: Scarecrow Press.

Liebowitz, J. 2009. *Knowledge Retention: Strategies and Solutions*. New York: Auerbach Publishing/Taylor & Francis.

Liebowitz, J., R. Bali, and N. Wickramasinghe, eds. 2007. Special issue on social networking and knowledge flows in organizations. *International Journal of Networking and Virtual Organizations*, 4(4).

Macdonald, M. 2003. Knowledge management in healthcare: What does it involve? How is it measured? *Healthcare Management Forum* 16(3).

Massoud, M.R., G.A. Nielsen, K. Nolan, T. Nolan, M.W. Schall, and C. Sevin. 2006. A framework for spread: From local improvements to system-wide change. IHI Innovation Series white paper. Institute for Healthcare Improvement, Cambridge, Mass. Available at www.IHI.org.

National Association of County and City Health Officials. 2006. 2005 National profile of local health departments. Washington, D.C.

National Association of County and City Health Officials. 2009. NACCHO survey of local health departments' budget cuts and workforce reductions. Available at http://www.naccho.org/advocacy/upload/report_lhdbudgets.pdf. Retrieved on Jan. 18, 2009.

Milstein, B. 2008. Hygeia's constellation: navigating health futures in a dynamic and democratic world. Syndemics Prevention Network, Centers for Disease Control and Prevention. Available at http://www.cdc.gov/syndemics/monograph/index.htm. Retrieved on Jan. 15, 2009.

Pablos, A. and R. Shademani. 2006. Knowledge translation in global health. *Journal of Continuing Education in the Health Professions* 26(1).

Palmer, J. 2009. Emergency 2.0 is coming to a website near you. *New Scientist*. Available at http://www.newscientist.com/article/mg19826545.900-emergency-20-is-coming-to-a-website-near-you.html?page=1. Retrieved Dec. 12, 2008.

Plaice, C. and P. Kitch. 2003. Embedding knowledge management in the NHS south-west: Pragmatic first steps for a practical concept. *Health Information and Libraries Journal* 20.

Revere, D., A. Turner, A. Madhavan, N. Rambo, P. Bugni, A. Kimball, and S. Fuller. 2007. Understanding the information needs of public health practitioners: A literature review to inform design of an interactive digital knowledge management system. *Journal of Biomedical Informatics*. 40.

Rolls, K., D. Kowal, D. Elliott, and A. Burrell. 2008. Building a statewide knowledge network for clinicians in intensive care units: Knowledge brokering and the NSW Intensive Care Coordination and Monitoring Unit ICCMU. *Australian Critical Care* 21.

Sanchez, M. and J. Cegarra. 2008. Implementing knowledge management practices in hospital-in-the-home units. *Journal of Nursing Care Quality* 23(1).

Shrader, K. 2006. Over 3,600 intelligence professionals tapping into "Intellipedia." Associated Press release. Available at http://www.usatoday.com/tech/news/techinnovations/2006-11-02-intellipedia_x.htm. Retrieved on Dec. 31, 2008.

Thamlikitkul, V. 2006. Bridging the gap between knowledge and action for health: Case studies. *Bulletin of the World Health Organization*, 84(8).

United Nations Foundation. 2007. Sustainable technology empowers healthcare delivery in Africa. Press release. Available at http://www.unfoundation.org/press-center/press-releases/2007/sustainable-technology-empowers-healthcare-in-Africa.html. Retrieved on Jan. 10, 2009.

UNAIDS. 2008. 2008 report on the global AIDS epidemic. World Health Organization. 2006. Taking stock: Health worker shortages and the response to AIDS. Available at http://www.unaids.org/en/KnowledgeCentre/HIVData/GlobalReport/2008/. Retrieved on Jan. 9, 2009.

United States President's Emergency Plan for AIDS Relief. 2007. Phones for health: Major public-private partnership to use mobile phones to fight HIV/AIDS pandemic. Press release. Available at http://www.pepfar.gov. Retrieved on Jan. 10, 2009.

World Health Organization. 2000. Smallpox. Available at http://www.who.int/mediacentre/factsheets/smallpox/en/. Retrieved on Jan. 20, 2009.

Chapter 3

Extending Cross-Generational Knowledge Flow Research in Edge Organizations*

Jay Liebowitz and Emil Ivanov

Contents

* This chapter was presented and published in the ICCRTS-13th Conference Proceedings, June 2008, DoD Command and Control Research Program, Seattle, WA (all rights are retained by the authors).

Acknowledgment

This research is sponsored in part by the Office of the Assistant Secretary of Defense for Networks and Information Integration, through its Command and Control Research Program and the Center for Edge Power at the Naval Postgraduate School. We greatly appreciate the support of Dr. Mark Nissen and Dr. David Alberts.

Introduction

Our previously funded edge research project (Liebowitz et al., 2007a) focused on cross-generational knowledge flows in edge organizations. An edge organization is network-centric and empowers decision making "on the edge," often relevant in public health situations. We found that cross-generational biases affect tacit knowledge transfer between edge-like teams. Our findings were based on the use of our university graduate capstone teams, whereby three to six individuals per team worked together on semester-long "real" projects. Our research was novel in that the combination of intergenerational differences (Wei, 2006; DiRomualdo, 2006), tacit knowledge transfer (Foos et al., 2006; Liebowitz, 2006a, 2006b, 2008, 2009; Nissen, 2006, 2007; Perrolle and Moris, 2007), and edge organizations (Alberts & Hayes, 2003, 2007) had never been studied.

One limitation of our research was the need to address how edge-like teams can overcome possible cross-generational biases in order to enhance knowledge flows for improved team productivity. Our prior research tested various hypotheses, but stopped just short of recommending ways to counter these intergenerational differences to stimulate team efficiency and effectiveness. Additionally, case studies in defense and industry need to be collected, analyzed, and discussed to show how edge-like teams have overcome difficulties resulting from cross-generational knowledge flows. The focus of our current research addresses these limitations.

Specifically, we first examine the field of ontologies to build an ontology for cross-generational knowledge flows in edge organizations. Once the ontology is built, the next step is to apply the ontology as a framework in order to determine types of knowledge and cross-generational knowledge flows that are critical to the success of edge organizations. A survey instrument can then be designed in order to identify these knowledge flows and knowledge gaps in three case studies. Social/organizational network analysis are then used to help identify, understand, and visualize these knowledge flows in order to provide recommendations on critical success factors for enabling cross-generational knowledge flows in edge organizations.

To date, the initial ontology for cross-generational knowledge flows in edge organizations has been constructed. Protégé, from Stanford University and the leading ontology development software tool, has been used to assist in this endeavor.

The survey instrument was developed, and the two edge-like case organizations used in our study are: U.S. Navy/defense—a Navy knowledge management team; and industry—an intelligent transportation system company's information technology team. The survey was sent out in early November 2007, and the responses were returned in December 2007. The responses were encoded, and social/organizational network analysis was applied using the social network analysis tool UCINET/NetDraw (http://www.analytictech.com).

Ontology Development for Cross-Generational Knowledge Flows in Edge Organizations

An ontology can be viewed as a semiformal model of a real-world domain which portrays that domain in terms of its most imperative concepts, as well as the interaction among them (Swartout and Tate, 1999). By creating an ontology for a domain, the developer endeavors to formalize the domain, explicitly listing the concepts (things) in that field and the way that they relate to one another.

The focal idea for building this ontology is to capture the main concepts and their interrelationships in the domain of cross-generational knowledge flows in edge organizations. To provide better integration with existing knowledge sources, we relied closely on the existing vocabulary and expressions available in both Liebowitz et al. (2007) and the key edge organization references (Alberts and Hayes, 2003, 2007).

Before we started building our ontology, we reviewed the best practices of ontology design principles and methodologies, as well as the available ontology development software tools. Ontology development could be equivalent with software engineering in complexity and principles of development. In the software engineering field, many matured methodologies already exist, such as rational unified process (Hunt, 2003) or extreme programming (Beck, 2000). Most of the ontology development authors (Gomez-Perez et al., 2004; Noy and McGuinness, 2001; Sure and Studer, 2002) recognize that the field of ontology development is not as mature as the field of software engineering, and presently there is no universal set of instituted and commonly accepted practices.

We followed the ontology methodology proposed by Noy and McGuinness (2001) for our ontology development. We carefully analyzed our key reference sources to look for important classes, instances, and relationships between terms. We used Protégé 3.1.1 (2007), developed by Stanford University, for the ontology development and encoding. Protégé provides visual interfaces for making classes, individuals, and properties, as well as an interface to test the ontology with different queries. It also provides support to generate graph diagrams that are almost intuitive and easy to understand. We created the ontology with its visual interface. Figure 3.1 shows the visual interface, which has different tabs.

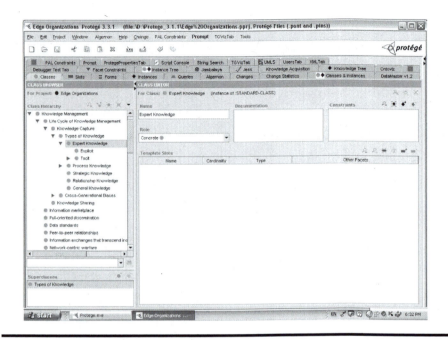

Figure 3.1 Screen shot of Protégé in the cross-generational knowledge flow in edge organization domain.

More tabs can be configured from the menu. The main tabs used are: "classes" (domain concepts) and their attributes and relationships; "properties" for creation of properties and setting their ranges or restrictions; and "individuals" for creation of instances in our data model. Jambalaya is a plug-in created for Protégé that visualizes regular Protégé and OWL knowledge bases. This visualization technique is designed to enhance browsing, exploring, and interaction with the knowledge structure. Figure 3.2 shows a view from our ontology with Jambalaya.

The resulting models (classes and instances) can be loaded and saved in various formats, including Extensible Markup Language (XML), Unified Modeling Language (UML), and Resource Description Framework (RDF). Protégé also provides a very scalable database back end. From a programmer's perspective, one of Protégé's most attractive features is that it provides an open source Application Programming Interface (API) to plug in Java components and access the domain models from its own application. As a result, systems can be developed very rapidly—starting with the underlying domain model, letting Protégé generate the basic user interface, and then gradually write widgets and plug-ins to customize its look and feel and behavior.

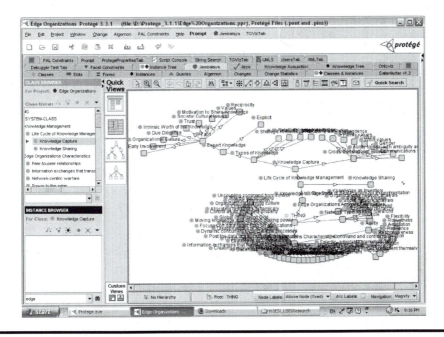

Figure 3.2   Screen shot using the Jambalaya plug-in for Protégé for our domain.

Analyzing Cross-Generational Knowledge Flows in Edge Organizations

Based on the ontology developed in the previous section, a survey instrument was developed to determine cross-generational knowledge flows in two edge-like case organizations (one in the military and one in industry). Social/organizational network analysis is being used to map these knowledge flows and knowledge gaps in the organizations. Liebowitz (2007), Liebowitz et al. (2007b), and Cross and Parker (2004) have written extensively about the importance of the informal organization and how innovation is increased through the informal social networks in organizations. Katzenbach Partners (2007) also echo these points in a recent report on "The Informal Organization." Clippinger (in press) reinforces the importance of social networks in edge organizations through leveraging trust and community building. Yoo et al. (2007) showed that knowledge sharing practices were enacted differently from the official strategy in order to close the post-merger knowledge gap. Even when looking across generations, a Generation Yer (or some call Generation Net) was quoted on the local news as saying that "my success depends upon my connections." Thus, social/organizational network analysis can be very useful to help map and visualize these cross-generational knowledge flows.

The survey instrument, derived from Liebowitz and Plexus Scientific Corp., contains the following questions as shown below:

A. Basic Demographics

1. Write your full name: _____

2. How long have you been working in your current organization? Please choose only one of the following:
   _____ Less than 1 year
   _____ 1–3 years
   _____ 4–6 years
   _____ 7–10 years
   _____ 11–15 years
   _____ 16 years or more

3. What is your primary role or function within the organization?
   _____

4. What generation were you born?
   _____ "War" generation (1945 or earlier)
   _____ Baby boomers (1946–1965)
   _____ Generation Xers (1966–1979)
   _____ Generation Yers (1980 or later)

5. How many years of professional experience do you possess?
   _____ Less than 1 year
   _____ 1–3 years
   _____ 4–6 years
   _____ 7–10 years
   _____ 11–15 years
   _____ 16 years or more

B. Team Characteristics ("Team" refers to your specific project/program team; if this doesn't apply, then kindly use "team" as department.)

1. Please respond to each of the following questions with a rating of 1–5.

```
Weak                                          Strong
 ├────────┼────────┼────────┼────────┤
 1        2        3        4        5
```

	Rating
a. How well do you rate your team's ability to work together with other teams?	

	Rating
b. How well do you rate your team's agility in terms of being well-suited to deal with uncertainty and unfamiliarity?	
c. How well is there a shared understanding of command intent among your team?	
d. How well do you rate your team's ability in terms of generating interactions between and among any and all team members?	
e. How well is there situational leadership on your team, whereby no single person will be in charge all the time?	
f. How well would you rate your team as being nonhierarchical?	
g. How well would you rate your team's degree of competency?	
h. How well would you rate your team's multitasking ability?	
i. How well do you rate your team's ability to utilize information technology via a robust network to facilitate information sharing?	
j. How well does your team exhibit strong work values among your team?	
k. How well does your team exhibit strong family values among your team?	
l. How well does your team exhibit strong communications flow among your team?	
m. How well does your team exhibit strong interpersonal trust among your team?	
n. What is the degree of cultural issues affecting your team?	
o. How well does your team encourage incentives to share knowledge?	
p. How well does your team exhibit reciprocity of knowledge shared among your team?	
q. How well does your team exhibit loyalty among members?	
r. What is the degree of gender issues affecting the team?	
s. What is the degree of cross-generational biases among the team?	

2. Please provide us with the name of each person (internal and external to your organization) with whom you interact in order to accomplish your tasks or assist him/her in accomplishing his/her tasks. Kindly mark "I" for internal person and "E" for external person. Please include their department/organization as well.

3. How long have you known this person?
   a = less than 1 year   d = 5–10 years
   b = 1–2 years   e = more than 10 years
   c = 3–5 years

4. Please indicate his/her hierarchical level within the organization relative to your own.
   a = higher than yours   b = equal to yours   c = lower than yours

5. Please indicate the frequency with which you interact with this person for information and collaboration purposes.
   a = seldom   c = often
   b = sometimes   d = very often

6. Who usually initiates the interaction?
   a = I generally initiate
   b = He/she generally initiates
   c = Equal amounts of initiation

7. Do you turn to this person for decision-making information, general information, or as a sounding board for ideas? Please indicate all that apply. (More than one answer may apply; e.g., D and S.)
   D = decision-making information   S = sounding board for ideas
   G = general information   O = other (please specify)

8. What topic(s) of information do you usually discuss with this person?

Survey Responses and Analysis

Two organizations were used for our cross-generational edge teams. The first was a Navy knowledge management team, and the second was an intelligent transportation system company IT team. We are looking at the following types of questions: (1) Does generation, tenure in the organization, and/or years of professional experience have an impact on the types of knowledge that are exchanged via cross-generational knowledge flows in edge organizations, in order for the organizations to meet their strategic objectives? (2) What factors suggest a successful cross-generational knowledge flow? (3) What factors are most important to an edge organization for promoting cross-generational knowledge flows? We have compiled the responses from the surveys in order to apply our social/organizational network analysis tool, UCINET/NetDraw (http://www.analytictech.com), to help analyze and visualize the cross-generational knowledge flows in these edge-like organizations (Liebowitz, 2007). This allows us to gather insight and recommend critical success factors for ensuring cross-generational knowledge flows in edge-like organizations.

According to the survey responses as shown in Figure 3.3 and Table 3.1, questions (a) through (i) relate to the characteristics of an edge organization. Questions (j) through (s) relate to characteristics of cross-generational knowledge flows. Interestingly, the average ratings from the team members of the case organizations show, within some slight varying degrees, that they possess the necessary characteristics of being an edge-like team. From Net's and Telv's respondents, some team members were positioned throughout the world with a cadre of team members being situated in the same area. In Net's and Telv's ratings, the only edge characteristic which was not fully satisfied was the team being nonhierarchical. In both cases, an average neutral response was indicated by the team respondents.

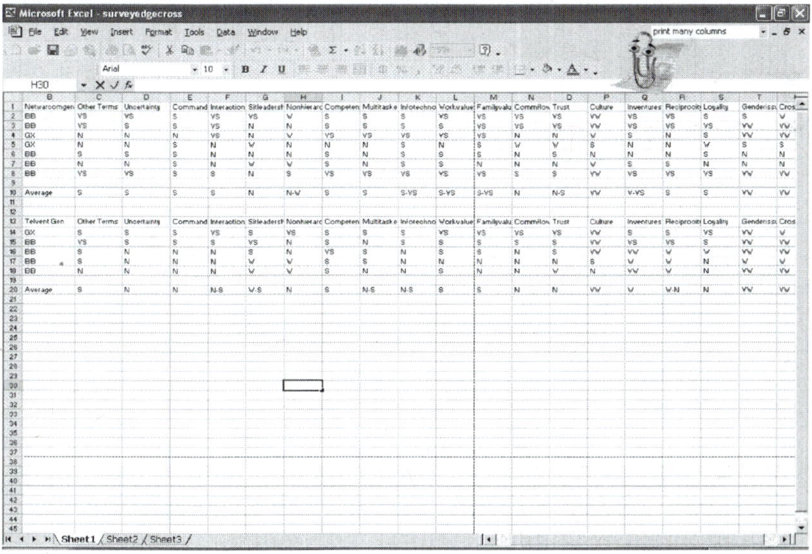

In terms of the survey respondents' average ratings dealing with cross-generational knowledge flows, questions (j) through (s) covered the main attributes based on Liebowitz et al. (2007). The average ratings generally showed that Net and Telv displayed the necessary characteristics for strong cross-generational knowledge flows within the team. However, there were some trust, reciprocity, and communications flow issues that existed, mostly with the Telv team, which could inhibit how successful the team would be in cross-generational knowledge flows.

Figure 3.3   Survey responses on team characteristics.

Table 3.1 Survey Average Ratings Relating to Team Characteristics

	Average Rating
a. How well do you rate your team's ability to work together with other teams?	Net: S Telv: S
b. How well do you rate your team's agility in terms of being well-suited to deal with uncertainty and unfamiliarity?	Net: S Telv: N
c. How well is there a shared understanding of command intent among your team?	Net: S Telv: N
d. How well do you rate your team's ability in terms of generating interactions between and among any and all team members?	Net: S Telv: N-S
e. How well is there situational leadership on your team, whereby no single person will be in charge all the time?	Net: N Telv: W-S
f. How well would you rate your team as being nonhierarchical?	Net: N-W Telv: N
g. How well would you rate your team's degree of competency?	Net: S Telv: S
h. How well would you rate your team's ability as being a good multitasker?	Net: S Telv: N-S
i. How well do you rate your team's ability to utilize information technology via a robust network to facilitate information sharing?	Net: S-VS Telv: N-S
j. How well does your team exhibit strong work values among your team?	Net: S-VS Telv: S
k. How well does your team exhibit strong family values among your team?	Net: S-VS Telv: S
l. How well does your team exhibit strong communications flow among your team?	Net: N Telv: N
m. How well does your team exhibit strong interpersonal trust among your team?	Net: N-S Telv: N
n. What is the degree of cultural issues affecting your team?	Net: VW Telv: VW
o. How well does your team encourage incentives to share knowledge?	Net: V-VS Telv: W
p. How well does your team exhibit reciprocity of knowledge shared among your team?	Net: S Tel: W-N

	Average Rating
q. How well does your team exhibit loyalty among members?	Net: S Telv: N
r. What is the degree of gender issues affecting your team?	Net: VW Telv: VW
s. What is the degree of cross-generational biases among your team?	Net: VW Telv: VW

In reviewing some of the literature on generational diversity as related to succession planning (Bedell, 2007), organizations must master the baby boomer–Generation X–Generation Y divide. In order to plan for the future, Bedell (2007) discusses some techniques in terms of ensuring better succession planning through involving the Generation Yers:

1. Onboarding: Take a cohort approach, connect their work, solicit their input, and have fun.
2. Training: Include Generation Xers and boomers with the Generation Yers in the training to heighten generational diversity awareness.
3. Mentoring/Reverse Mentoring: Match a Generation Yer with a boomer, and let Generation Yer be a "technology mentor."
4. Coaching: Coach the team at the beginning and beyond.
5. Give Them a Seat at the Table: Get the Generation Yer involved so he or she can contribute to the decision-making process.
6. Passport Initiatives: Let the Generation Yer "travel" to different functional and geographical areas within the company to bridge across the silos.

Multidimensional analysis portrays the clusters of interactions among the team members. For the Net team, people do not stick with only their "generational" colleagues. The same held true based on the years of professional experience—that is, the team members did not just stay with those who had the same years of professional experience as they did.

In analyzing the Net team further, the generational issues were nonapparent in terms of who they contact, the relationship with that individual, the level within the team, the frequency of contact, the initiator of the contact, and the information type sought. The average responses for the Net team were: contacted person's relationship was less than one year, lower level in the organization, often or very often frequency of contact, equal or self-initiated contacts, and decision-making and general types of information sought.

Spring embedding can be used to position the network actors based on their geodesic distances and to analyze the direction and strength of the knowledge flows in the network (Polites and Watson, 2008). Figure 3.4 shows spring embedding of the Net team by generation, and clusters begin to emerge, as well as connections between the clusters. The BB refers to baby boomer, the GX refers to Generation Xer, and the P refers to a Person Contact. BB2, BB5, and GX2 are "cutpoints," meaning that these network members emerge if the network is cut into loosely coupled components. These individuals could be knowledge enablers, but also could play the role of knowledge inhibitors if wanted. Thus, the knowledge flows can be affected by these individuals. If you convert the P to its appropriate generation, as shown in Figure 3.5, some interesting results appear. Most of the people contacted for advice were baby boomers. However, cross-generational knowledge flows take place between the baby boomers and the Generation Xers, as shown by GX1 and GX2 contacting the BB, and BB1 and BB2 contacting the GX, and BB2, BB3, BB4, and BB5 contacting the BB.

In analyzing the Telv team, the team members were either baby boomers or Generation Xers. The boomers had either seven to ten years of professional experience or eleven to fifteen years. The Generation Xers had four to six years of professional experience. The boomers on the team sought out people who had more years of experience (typically five to ten years) than those sought out by the Generation Xers (one to two years). This is not unusual, as the boomers had been working at Telv

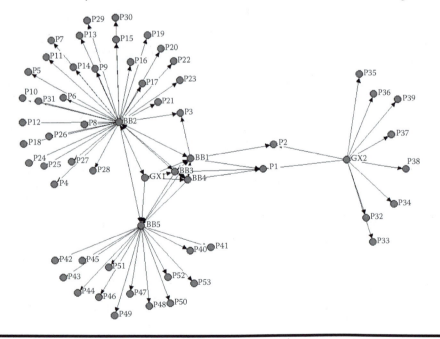

Figure 3.4   Net team layout by generation (spring embedding).

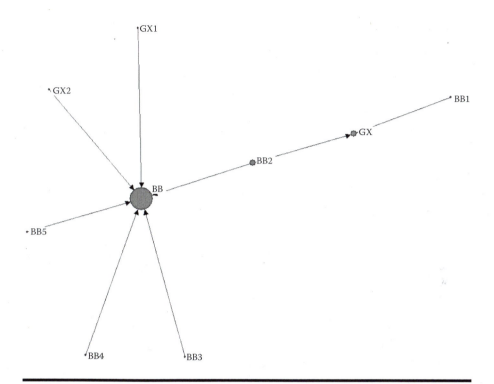

Figure 3.5   Net team (degree of centrality) by converting all nodes to generations.

longer than the Generation Xers and had developed longer relationships over those years. Figure 3.6 shows the reciprocal ties (lighter lines) and the nonreciprocal ties (darker lines) between the Telv team members and their contacts in terms of years of professional experience. The larger square shows a higher degree of centrality.

Figure 3.7 shows the Telv team in terms of betweenness centrality. Here, BB2 and GX1 have the highest values for betweenness—that is, they are the most sought after "go-betweens" within the Telv team. Figure 3.8 indicates the connections between the Telv team members and those they reach out to for advice based on the number of years they know them.

In looking across the two generations on the team, there was not a difference in the hierarchy of those contacted (equal), the frequency of those contacted (often), or the initiator of those contacts (the other person usually initiates). The only slight difference between the two generations on the Telv team was that the boomers with seven to ten years of professional experience sought out information for decision making and general purposes, whereas the boomers with eleven to fifteen years of experience and the Generation Xers sought out people for decision-making, general, and sounding board types of information.

In order to determine how successful the cross-generational knowledge flows are within the teams, we must associate them with the knowledge management (KM)

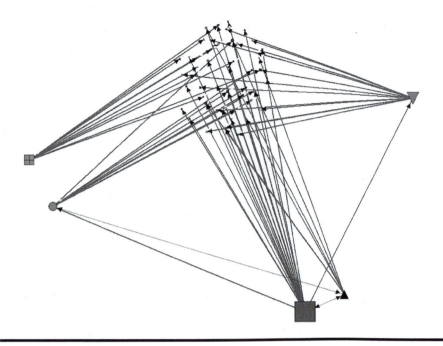

Figure 3.6 Telv team and its contacts in terms of years of professional experience.

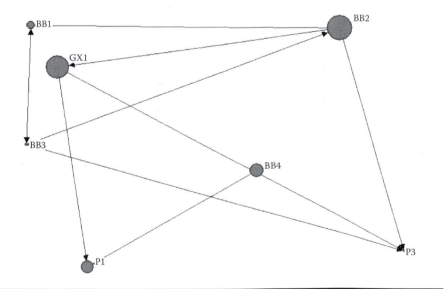

Figure 3.7 Telv team betweenness centrality.

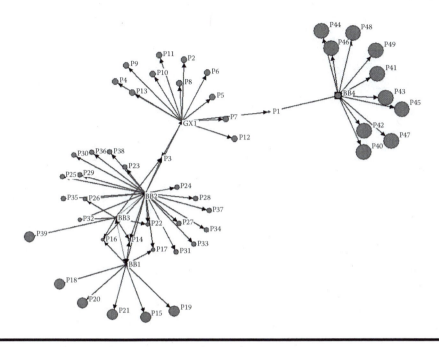

Figure 3.8 Telv team relationship length.

strategic goals of the team. The strategic goals related to knowledge management deal with five categories: adaptability/agility (AA), creativity/innovation (C), institutional memory building (IM), organizational internal effectiveness (IE), and organizational external effectiveness (EE). For example, Telv's adaptability goal is to rapidly commercialize new products and services, and its institutional memory building goal is to retain critical knowledge before the individual leaves. We associated the specific knowledge topics indicated by the survey respondents with the five strategic KM goals. Then, we examined the knowledge flows across generations by individual and department/function as related to the knowledge topics and knowledge types. In this manner, we can see if there are any structural holes or knowledge gaps in terms of the cross-generational knowledge flows as contributing to the team's KM goals.

The spring-embedded view of the Telv team, as shown in Figure 3.9, shows that the Systems Engineering department is the liaison between BB1 and BB3; GX1 is the liaison within the IT outsourced group in India; and BB4 (the team leader) has direct ties to senior management in the U.S. and India. Probing deeper to examine the individuals by knowledge topic (Infotopic) and knowledge type (Infotype), Figures 3.10 and 3.11 show that the greatest connections among the Telv team individuals are with adaptability/agility (AA), creativity (C), organizational internal

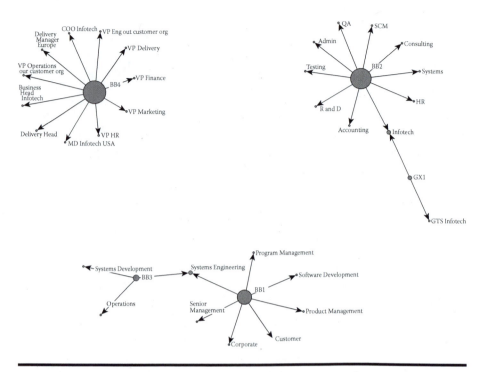

Figure 3.9   Telv team organizational department contacts (spring embedding).

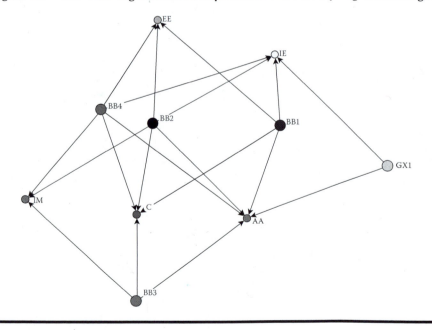

Figure 3.10   Telv team ID versus infotopic.

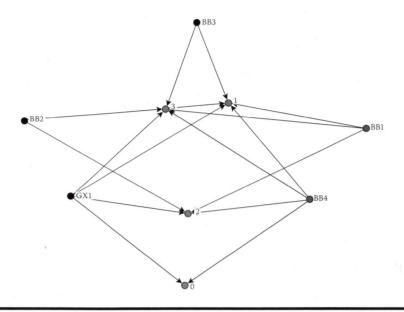

Figure 3.11   Telv team ID versus infotype.

effectiveness (IE), and organizational external effectiveness (EE). In addition, most of the individuals reach out to others in the Telv team for first, decision-making information (denoted by the number 3 in Figure 3.11), and then general information (denoted by the number 1) and sounding-board information (denoted by number 2; other information is denoted by 0).

In looking across the organizational units on the Telv team by knowledge topic and knowledge type, Figures 3.12 and 3.13 show the following: Organizational internal effectiveness (IE) has the highest number of direct ties with the departments and thus is a high priority; the human resources (HR) and consulting departments have the highest closeness values related to institutional nemory (IM); and organizational internal effectiveness (IE) possesses the highest betweenness value followed by adaptability/agility (AA). Also, the senior management members, as expected, have the closest ties to the decision-making information (denoted by the number 3 in Figure 3.13).

Returning to our original research questions, what can we learn from these case studies? Does generation, tenure in the organization, or years of professional experience have an impact on the types of knowledge that are exchanged via cross-generational knowledge flows in edge organizations, in order for the organizations to meet their strategic objectives? From our exploratory case studies using the Net and Telv teams, we found that information flow networks are formed by knowledge sharing within the teams, especially the geographically distributed team like the Net team. Organizational adaptability is a function of the ability to learn and to act due to shifting events (Leinonen and Bluemink, 2008; Anantatmula, 2007;

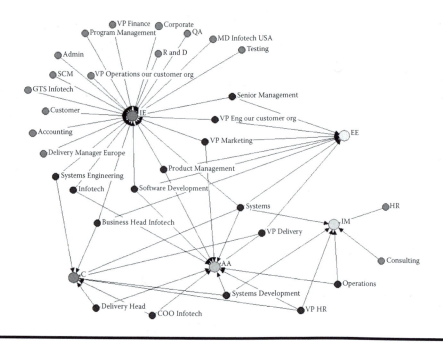

Figure 3.12 Telv team organizational department versus infotopic.

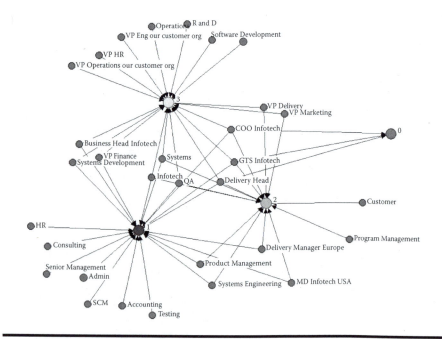

Figure 3.13 Telv team organizational department versus infotype.

Tseng, 2008; Courtney et al., 2007). On the other hand, agility is the speed of response to potential changes. The baby boomers in both studied groups act as power networks, as they are directly linked to the leadership. They are the actors who invigorate others. Betweenness, as to the extent in which a particular actor is measured against (position) various other actors in the network, are again the baby boomers. Cross and Parker (2004) state that actors with high betweenness and those who are closely connected to them become high performers as well. For this reason, high energy tends to gather in discernible pockets within an organization and, in our case studies, is more visible in the Net team.

Edge organizations highlight a degree of independence of the units. They are flexible, allowing teams to be set up in response to new tasks. The results of the surveys and our social network analysis suggest that resourcefulness can enhance the performance of people for a variety of tasks, including decision making. Another characteristic of the edge organization is situational awareness (SA), which is about being aware of what is going on. Both teams indicated that internal and external effectiveness and institutional memory are among the categories for sharing and transferring knowledge. These categories are tightly linked to SA as well. The years of professional experience in baby boomers are strongly related with SA. From a recent experimental study (Marks et al., 2008), knowledge sharing was found to be facilitated by management's reminders of the importance of the goal and reminders about rivals. In the same study, knowledge sharing was more likely to occur with individuals with prosocial traits—that is, people concerned more about the group's collective goals versus individual agendas. In our case studies, we would need to further study the prosocial nature of the individuals among the teams.

In addressing the other two research questions, and based on the exploratory case studies, the following were important as critical success factors for cross-generational knowledge flows: shared understanding, reciprocity, intrinsic worth of the knowledge, subset of overlapping values to reduce generational gaps, convenient knowledge transfer mechanisms, and established trust/rapport. Shared understanding refers to having a mutual conveyance and agreement of ideas that are shared between two parties. Reciprocity refers to being willing to share one's knowledge, because given a similar situation, the knowledge recipient would in turn share his or her knowledge with the individual. Intrinsic worth of knowledge refers to the value and merit of the knowledge being conveyed. A subset of overlapping values to reduce generational gaps also is important to lead to a common, shared understanding. Convenient knowledge transfer mechanisms need to exist for cross-generational knowledge flows so that "user adoption" will be enhanced. These knowledge transfer mechanisms could be either codified or personalized approaches to sharing knowledge. Last, having interpersonal trust and respect for each other will enhance knowledge sharing as well.

Curiously enough, these critical success factors are not unique to just cross-generational knowledge flows. Most of the literature on knowledge management performance or success (Guo and Sheffield, 2008) highlights many of these factors. Interestingly too, the critical success factors for cross-generational knowledge flows in edge organizations, as exemplified in our two case studies, also reflect the same set of success factors with two caveats. The first caveat deals with establishing trust and rapport among the team members. This is especially important in edge organizations due to situational leadership, whereby the leadership changes based on the task at hand and the team leader may rotate according to the necessary set of skills and competencies needed for a given mission. The second caveat deals with having convenient knowledge transfer mechanisms. In an edge organization, network centricity is a common factor; therefore, this should help provide convenient knowledge transfer mechanisms among the team.

In looking ahead toward the future, research in cross-generational knowledge flows, particularly in the context of edge organizations, is fertile ground. This is especially true in today's environment where knowledge retention issues loom over many organizations. Our exploratory case study approach is limited and generalizability may be difficult to attain due to the inherit qualities of the case study method. However, we believe our research confirms many of the hypotheses from our earlier research (Liebowitz et al., 2007)

Summary

With human capital strategy issues looming in many organizations, it becomes increasingly important to best leverage knowledge internally and externally for organizations to succeed. Furthermore, for organizations to be more adaptive and agile, especially in the case of edge organizations, fluid knowledge flows become even more paramount. Cross-generational knowledge flow in edge organizations is an exciting area of research that has been partly overlooked. This paper sheds some additional light on this topic by extending our previous research through the use of ontologies and social/organizational network analysis applied to real cases in defense and industry.

References

Alberts, D.S. and R.E. Hayes (2003). Power to the edge: Command and control in the information age, U.S. Department of Defense (DoD) Command and Control Research Program, Washington, D.C., http://www.dodccrp.org.

Alberts, D.S. and R.E. Hayes (2007). Planning complex endeavors, DoD Command and Control Research Program, Washington, D.C., http://www.dodccrp.org.

Anantatmula, V. (2007). Linking KM effectiveness attributes to organizational performance, *VINE: The Journal of Information and Knowledge Management Systems*, 37, 2.

Beck. K. (2000). *Extreme Programming Explained: Embrace Change*, Addison-Wesley. Reading, MA.

Bedell, K. (2007). Succession planning: Generational diversity, *Talent Management Magazine*, December.

Clippinger, J. (in press). Chapter five, Human nature and social networks, http://www.social-physics.org/images/Human_Nature.pdf.

Courtney, H., E. Navarro, and C. O'Hare (2007). The dynamic organic transformational team model for high-performance knowledge worker teams, *Team Performance Management Journal*, 13, 1 and 2.

Cross, R. and A. Parker (2004). *The Hidden Power of Social Networks*, Harvard Business School Press, Cambridge, MA.

DiRomualdo, T. (2006). Viewpoint: Geezers, crungers, GenXers, and geeks: A look at workplace generational conflict, *Journal of Financial Planning*, October.

Foos, T., G. Schum, and S. Rothenberg (2006). Tacit knowledge transfer and the knowledge disconnect, *Journal of Knowledge Management*, 10, 1, 6–18.

Gomez-Perez A., M. Fernandez-Lopez, and O. Corcho (2004). Ontological engineering with examples from the areas of knowledge management, e-commerce and the semantic Web, *Advanced Information and Knowledge Processing*.

Guo, Z. and J. Sheffield (2008). A paradigmatic and methodological examination of knowledge management research: 2000 to 2004, *Decision Support Systems Journal*, 44, February.

Hunt. J. (2003). Guide to the unified process featuring UML, Java and Design patterns, *Springer Professional Computing*, September.

Katzenbach Partners (2007). *The Informal Organization*, New York.

Leinonen, P. and J. Bluemink (2008). The distributed team members' explanations of knowledge they assume to be ahared, *Journal of Workplace Learning*, 20, 1.

Liebowitz, J. (2006a). *What They Didn't Tell You About Knowledge Management*, Scarecrow Press/Rowman & Littlefield, Lanham, Md.

Liebowitz, J. (2006b). *Strategic Intelligence: Business Intelligence, Competitive Intelligence, and Knowledge Management*, Auerbach Publishing/Taylor & Francis, New York.

Liebowitz, J. (2007). *Social Networking: The Essence of Innovation*, Scarecrow Press/Rowman & Littlefield, Lanham, Md.

Liebowitz, J., Ed. (2008). *Making Cents Out of Knowledge Management*, Scarecrow Press/Rowman & Littlefield, Lanham, Md.

Liebowitz, J. (2009). *Knowledge Retention: Strategies and Solutions*, Auerbach Publishing/Taylor & Francis, New York.

Liebowitz, J., N. Ayyavoo, H. Nguyen, D. Carran, and J. Simien (2007). Cross-generational knowledge flows in edge organizations, *Industrial Management & Data Systems Journal*, 107, 2.

Liebowitz, J., R. Bali, and N. Wickramasinghe, Eds. (2007). Special issue on social networking and knowledge flows in organizations, *International Journal of Networking and Virtual Organizations*, 4, 4.

Marks, P., P. Polak, S. McCoy, and D. Galletta (2008). Sharing knowledge, *Communications of the ACM*, 51, 2, February.

Nissen, M.E. (2006). *Harnessing Knowledge Dynamics*, IRM Press, Hershey, PA.

Nissen, M.E. (2007). Enhancing organizational metacognition: Flow visualization to make the knowledge network explicit, *International Journal on Networking and Virtual Organizations*, 4, 4.

Noy, N.F. and D. McGuinness (2001). Ontology development 101: A guide to creating your first ontology, technical report KSL-01-05 and SMI-2001-0880, Stanford Knowledge Systems Laboratory and Stanford Medical Informatics, Palo Alto, CA.

Perrolle, P. and F. Moris (2007). Advancing measures of innovation: Knowledge flows, business metrics, and measurement strategies, National Science Foundation, workshop report NSF 07-306, Washington, D.C.

Polites, G. and R. Watson (2008). The centrality and prestige of CACM, *Communications of the ACM*, 51, 1.

Protégé editor 3.3.1, available at http://protege.stanford.edu, accessed on Nov. 15, 2007.

Sure Y. and R. Studer (2002). On-to-knowledge methodology, on-to-knowledge deliverable 18, AIFB, University of Karlsruhe, available at http://www.aifb.unikarlsruhe.de/WBS/ysu/publications/OTK-D18 v1-0.pdf.

Swartout, W. and A. Tate (1999). Ontologies: Guest editors' introduction, *IEEE Intelligent Systems*, special issue on ontologies, 14, 1, (Jan./Feb.), 18–19.

Tseng, S.M. (2008). Knowledge management system performance measure index, *Expert Systems With Applications: An International Journal*, Elsevier 34.

Wei, K. (2006). Understanding the impact of national cultural difference on knowledge sharing process in global virtual teams, The 5th Annual Knowledge Management Doctoral Consortium, presented at Queen's University, Kingston, Canada.

Yoo, Y., K. Lyytinen, and D. Heo (2007). Closing the gap: Towards a process model of post-merger knowledge sharing, *Information Systems Journal*, 17.

Chapter 4

Knowledge Retention Trends and Strategies for Knowledge Workers and Organizations

Masud Cader and Jay Liebowitz

Contents

Introduction

A confluence of trends is beginning to change the way organizations and countries treat their most critical knowledge and people with the skills to use specialized knowledge:

- Aging "baby boomer" demographic trends in the U.S. and other developed countries
- Increased migration of experienced specialist workers (e.g., nurses) from less-developed countries to developed countries
- Globalization of services
- Low pipeline replenishment rates contribute to the need for retaining knowledge at organizational and national levels

Recent contrary trends suggest lower urgency for retaining knowledge of U.S. workers: A worsening economic situation and higher life expectancy likely will delay retirement and extend working life. The worsening economic situation precipitated by the "credit crunch" contagion has negatively impacted retirement wealth in terms of falling house values and diminished pension benefits available to retirees. Financial uncertainty will cause potential retirees to postpone early retirement, and perhaps push traditional retirement age to sixty-seven or beyond (Losey, 2008).

This easing in urgency may be a temporary blip. Demographic trends are likely to bring organizational knowledge retention to the fore at most government and commercial organizations in the next decade. An increasing U.S. population dependency ratio caused by the impending retirement of baby boomers is a key risk to organizations in the coming twenty years—a risk that is perhaps not fully recognized by management. Organizational knowledge retention can affect operational levels, and when critical, may impact ability to implement strategy (Liebowitz, 2009). In extreme cases, future earnings and the viability of the organization itself are impacted (De Long and Davenport, 2003).

The baby boomer generation is currently reaching retirement (Ebrahimi, Saives, and Holford, 2008), while knowledge workers are increasingly key to filling the fastest-growing jobs of the future (Lord and Farrington, 2006). Baby boomers will probably retire at an increasing rate (Inman and Inman, 2004), taking with them knowledge that is crucial to existing operations and innovation (Liebowitz and Liebowitz, 2006), although some may postpone retirement, leading to intergenerational workforce challenges (Lord and Farrington, 2006). All these trends could mean "a shortage of 10 million workers by 2010" (Inman and Inman, 2004).

Globalization of services means that migration of skilled employees from less-developed countries is increasingly relied upon to fill gaps, as "about 65% of all economically active migrants . . . are classed as highly skilled" (Stillwell et al., 2004). Outsourcing—a short-term solution to brain drain—perpetuates "the revolving door" as "employees are no longer making long term commitments to companies and companies are no longer making long term commitments to employees as evidenced by outsourcing internal jobs" (McManus et al., 2003). The U.S. federal government is depending more and more on outsourcing to private companies for information technology (IT) and specialized functions, so much so that the number of private federal contractors has now risen to 7.5 million, which is four times greater than the federal workforce itself, according to the report. Such a trend is leading the government to the "outsourcing (of) its brain" (Rawstory, 2007; Wysocki, 2007).

Migration of skilled labor is reaching epidemic proportions in some regions. For example, 1 in 37 in the Caribbean has migrated, and roughly two-thirds of Jamaica's nursing population has already emigrated. Nurses predominately emigrate to the U.S., U.K., and other developed countries, where the demand–pull is strong. The U.S. nurse ratio is 97 per 10,000 people, while in the Caribbean region, where HIV/AIDS prevalence is second only to sub-Saharan Africa, the nurse ratio ranges are at best from just over 50 (Barbados and Cayman Islands) to a low of 1.1 in Haiti. In a large population center of Jamaica the rate is 17, while in relatively affluent Trinidad the rate stands at only 29 (Salmon et al., 2007).

In a recent strategy report the International Finance Corp. (IFC—A World Bank Group) (IFC, 2008a) proposed a health policy strategy in Africa of formally facilitating, "public-private partnerships [PPPs] with governments aimed at leveraging the capacities of the private sector to improve the volume of medical professionals trained, e.g., could include interventions to create sufficient volumes for domestic and 'export' purposes as in Philippines and Thailand." One example of PPPs is the Managed Migration Program of the Caribbean that is a "regional strategy for retaining an adequate number of competent nursing personnel to deliver health programs and services to the Caribbean nationals." This coordinating network of private and public entities is focused on terms and conditions of work, recruitment, retention and training, value of nursing, utilization and deployment, management practices, including succession planning, and policy development (Salmon et al., 2007).

Trends suggest that knowledge retention will become increasingly more important for governments and organizations. Appropriate policies and coordination among interested parties—nongovernmental, multilaterals, and government organizations at all levels—are critical to balancing the needs of developed and developing countries with experienced staff and simultaneously preserving rights of citizens to practice nursing or other professions in other countries.

Organizational knowledge retention is primarily about preserving the organization's ability to use specialized and critical knowledge in achieving objectives. According to Frigo (2006), it consists of understanding the existing position in the firm, focusing on policies to identify and retain the right people, and transcending organizational policies.

Another view is that knowledge is represented by the network of collaborations and relationships among knowledge workers (whether intraorganization or interorganizational). Lintern et al. (2002) suggest that "explicit knowledge tends to be individual but implicit knowledge is shared." In this context, Lintern et al. (2002) say that we should not talk about "retention but continuity."

The results discussed in this paper focus on knowledge retention from employee perspectives. Other surveys (Monster, 2007) tend to survey human resource (HR) professionals at organizations—thus deriving an organizational perspective of knowledge retention, while others studied small, homogeneous samples (Philip and Turnbull, 2006). The result of applying a nineteen-question survey instrument, open to the general public, is used to explore perceptions of knowledge retention from sixty-nine respondents. A materially similar survey was directed at a sample of IFC sector specialists and is examined qualitatively due to the small sample properties of an additional eleven respondents.

Literature Overview and Survey Variables

It is no surprise that knowledge workers are relatively reluctant to share expertise and underlying knowledge, although motivations will differ (De Long, 2005). Lahti and Beyerlein (2000) found that "knowledge is still power...so this causes one to be more cautious....If you transfer too much knowledge to clients, they may not need you in the future." Liebowitz and Liebowitz (2006) also described a Georgetown University administrator who wanted to "reduce the institutional dependence on specialized personnel with 'secret knowledge' that allows them to complete tasks nobody else can perform." De Long and Davenport (2003) described Siemens' practice as including the "expert's level of motivation and capability for sharing the knowledge."

Lee and Maurer (1997) state that there are five general characteristics of professionals in high-tech firms: "First, they are expert in some abstract knowledge base that was acquired over a long period of time. Second, these professionals perceive a basic right to work in an autonomous fashion. Third, these knowledge workers identify with their chosen profession and other members of that profession. Fourth, they hold an ethically based responsibility to help their clients (or employers). Fifth, knowledge workers value a collective standard (i.e., code of professional conduct and feel committed to enforcement of that standard)."

The intangible nature of knowledge makes it more difficult to manage. While a knowledge management (KM) "lessons learned" system may allow for stores of expert interviews and cases, the problem is about motivating remaining staff to invest time learning from case databases and videotaped interviews (De Long, 2005). Hesketh (1997) says that, "maximizing the chance of developing transferable expertise involves combining elements of rule-based and exemplar-based learning, it also requires a lengthening of the time during skill acquisition when analytical processing is involved." A number of authors suggest that the more tacit the knowledge the more appropriate it is to transfer knowledge using mentoring techniques. Hesketh (1997) describes lifting the novice to a "routine expert" and finally to an "adaptive expert" using "situated learning techniques" as well as "extended practice." In essence, the problem with expertise is that the more one is an expert, the more difficult it is to codify the tacit knowledge and transfer the expertise to another, especially under tight succession deadlines.

De Long and Davenport (2003) and Liebowitz (2003) suggest a number of techniques for retaining knowledge, including more proactive monitoring of potential expert turnover, assessment of knowledge criticality, and knowledge gaps. Liebowitz (2003) goes further in directing primary experts to formally mentor individuals who are receptive and able to learn and develop the expertise at risk, but Szulanski (1996) describes three barriers, including "absorptive capacity" of the recipient, "causal ambiguity" regarding recipient understanding of cause-and-effect relationships, and quality of the relationship between mentor and recipient. On the policy level, Liebowitz (2003) asserts that the government's strategy for record retention should be broadened, and HR enablers should provide recognition (formal and informal) through performance management and devices such as "recognition days." Formal facilitators of knowledge management also should be involved in embedding key KM and record management steps into daily business processes, and in the associated change management to make the changes meaningful and assure linkage of knowledge retention, sharing, and management to work processes rewarded under existing HR policies. Lahti and Beyerlein (2000) describe a similar schema:

- Refine compensation systems to provide an incentive for sharing knowledge.
- Revise performance management systems to make individuals accountable for transferring knowledge.
- Use organizational structures that encourage collaboration and knowledge transfer.
- Develop a knowledge vision and strategy and align them with organizational systems to assist in developing a knowledge-sharing culture.
- Devise and implement the appropriate combination of knowledge repositories and informal knowledge transfer mechanisms (networks of individuals, peer coaching) in accordance with the knowledge strategy.
- Model knowledge-sharing behavior at the management level.

Ray and Snyder (2006) nicely sum up a retention strategy as a synthesis of four approaches, including human resource management, automation, recording, and education.

There are contrary views on the utility of knowledge management in general, and in regard to the "importance of forgetting" (Monkey, 2005). Wilson (2002) presents a contrarian view of knowledge management. He writes, "'knowledge management' idea is, in large part, a management fad promulgated mainly by certain consultancy companies, and the probability is that it will fade away like previous fads. It rests on two foundations: the management of information—where a large part of the fad exists (and where the 'search and replace marketing' phenomenon is found), and the effective management of work practices. However, these latter practices are predicated upon a Utopian idea of organizational culture in which the benefits of information exchange are shared by all, where individuals are given autonomy in the development of their expertise, and where 'communities' within the organization can determine how that expertise will be used."

Knowledge Retention Survey Methodology

The knowledge retention survey (Liebowitz, 2008) was designed to capture nineteen questions regarding perception and attitudes toward organizational knowledge retention. The survey recorded demographic information, knowledge criticality, transfer mechanisms, job profile activities, and constraints faced in retention and sharing.

The following was used to conduct the survey:

1. The survey was hosted on surveymonkey.com and accessible through a secure URL (https protocol).
2. The survey was distributed in paper form to conference participants and selected special-interest groups.
3. The Web-based survey was announced through knowledge management blogs and KM-related Listservs.
4. The survey was open electronically from April 22 through May 29, 2008.
5. The survey responses were collected into Excel from both paper and online sources.
6. The results were presented in summary form and disallowed individual participant identification.

Analysis of Knowledge Retention Survey

Respondents were from a diverse group of companies, with the majority from the service industry. Sixty-nine people responded to the survey. Sixty-four people cited forty-two unique employer institutions, and five remained anonymous. Of the forty-two institutions, twenty-one were commercial, four tertiary education, fourteen governmental (one Canadian and thirteen U.S.), and three not-for-profit organizations based on names and e-mail top-level domains. Internet top-level domains are not an extremely reliable classification system, so NAICS[1] was adopted for detailed analysis.

Main activities of the forty-two organizations were classified according to the NAICS* primary-level codes as reported in financial or other regulatory or government reports (see Figure 4.1). Thirty-two percent of the identified sample firms were professional, scientific, and technical services, and 14% were health care and social assistance followed by administrative and support (9%). Manufacturing

---

* NAICS is a hierarchical industry classification system used by statistical agencies of the United States for classifying business establishments. NAICS includes 1,170 industries, of which 565 are service-based industries.

Business Type of Entity
(62 respondents from 42 organizations)

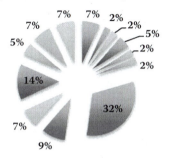

- Manufacturing
- Retail Trade
- Finance and Insurance
- Professional, Scientific, and Technical Services
- Educational Services
- Accommodation and Food Services
- Unclassified

- Wholesale Trade
- Information
- Real Estate and Rental and Leasing
- Administrative and Support
- Health Care and Social Assistance
- Other Services (excludes Public Administration)

Figure 4.1   Sixty-two of 69 respondents identified 42 employers allowing sector classification based on North American Industry Classification Code scheme. The majority of identified institutions were classified professional, scientific, and technical services, or health care and social assistance.

(7%), wholesale trade (2%), and retail trade (2%) comprised a smaller proportion than expected in a true random sample, as did finance-related (2%) and real estate (2%). This was an artifact of the convenience sample, and the fact that knowledge-management venues and promotion outlets were primarily used to market and thus drive the sample.

Respondent organizations are large and U.S. headquartered. Eighty-eight percent of the sample answering indicated their organizations were headquartered in the U.S., 7% in Europe, 3% in Canada, and the remaining 1% in another region. Organizations were generally large institutions with 56% from organizations with more than 150 employees, and 44% with 15 or fewer employees (see Figure 4.2). The U.S. federal government and the government of Quebec were among the largest employers, while EDS was an example of a large private-sector employer.

An unclear relationship was found between years to retirement or leaving the organization and tenure of employment in the organization. The expected correlation between longer tenure at an organization and planned time to retirement or leaving the organization did not materialize. Of the six respondents with a twenty-plus-year tenure, four expected to retire in two to five years, but none immediately, one provided no response, and another had no plan.

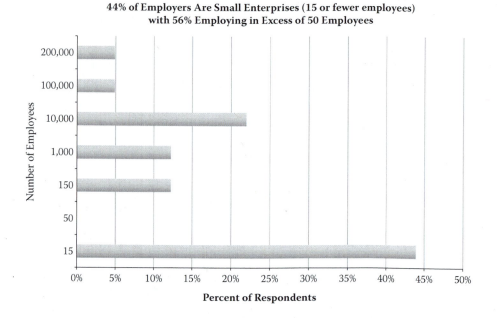

**44% of Employers Are Small Enterprises (15 or fewer employees)
with 56% Employing in Excess of 50 Employees**

Figure 4.2 Most respondents identifying their companies are employed by large organizations. However, a significant 44% of employers are small enterprises.

Other categories were much noisier (i.e., low correlation): For the thirteen respondents who have been with their organization for more than a decade but less than twenty years, only two expected to retire or leave within the next five years, six expected to retire or leave in six to ten years, one in eleven to twenty years, three had no plan, and one never planned to retire.

Length of service is relatively short among respondents (see Figure 4.3). The sample proved to be an adequate cross-section, with 41% of respondents having five or fewer years of service to their current employer, signifying a relatively low chance that the sample was biased to baby boomers. An additional 30% had service of six to ten years, and 28% had more than a decade of service.

Most will not retire or leave their organization soon (see Figure 4.4). Less than one-third of the sample answering indicated their expectation to either retire or leave their current employer organization within five years. Other surveys tend to yield even higher rates; for example, 80% of HR managers said that 30% of their staff would be eligible for retirement within the next ten years (Monster, 2007).

Survey respondents were asked to identify and describe self-perception of their critical knowledge area or expertise, and to rate how strategic the knowledge was

Forty-one Percent of Respondents Have 5 or Fewer years
of Service to Current Employer

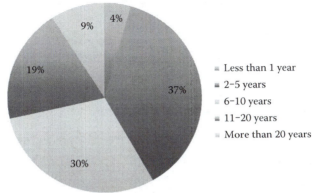

Figure 4.3   No clear baby boomer bias in the sample. Forty-one percent of respondents had 5 or less years of service to the current employer and 28% had more than 10 years of service to the current employer.

Fewer than 30% of Respondents Plan to Retire
or Leave Present Employer Within the Next 5 Years

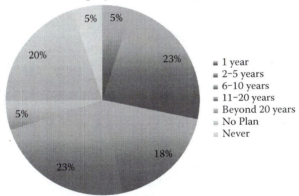

Figure 4.4   Forty-three percent would plan to leave or retire within the next decade. In some fields engineers generally leave at 50, so extending retirement age may not be too effective (Kennedy, 2006) as a retention strategy. Estimates tend to vary substantially: "Roughly 60% of experienced managers will retire by 2010" (Parise et al., 2006), while 28% of direct employment in the nuclear power generation sector will retire within five years (Ray and Snyder, 2006).

relative to the strategic mission and vision of the organization. Together these two elements gave an indication of the criticality of knowledge at risk. The expectation was that people with more critical knowledge would likely have a backup expert in the organization and have been subject to formal retention strategies, assuring continuity and retention, as well as reducing operational risk.

Critical expertise was dominated by specialized domain-specific knowledge (see Table 4.1). Just more than 22% of the sample identified their critical expertise as being in niche areas (biomedical, war on terror, etc.), 19% offered their expertise in KM or KM-related areas, including social network and "connecting the dots" expertise. Twelve percent expressed process-related expertise, and another 12% sales and relationship management knowledge.

Most respondents (more than 60%) believe that their knowledge is critical to the organization—not merely at a tactical level, but at the level of the organization's strategic mission and vision.

The Monster (2007) survey of HR officers at 550 firms finds that most respondents (77%) do not have a formal method to identify an organization's critical knowledge. The latter result is suggestive that employee self-perception and HR representatives' views on criticality of an employee's knowledge are likely not similar.

Critical knowledge should be retained (see Figure 4.5). The survey asked about the existence of an organization's knowledge retention strategy, including the existence of a backup, and the transfer mechanisms most and least frequently used.

Table 4.1 Critical Knowledge Classification Based on Qualitative Coding of Free-Text Responses Describing Respondent Job Family

Critical Knowledge/Expertise Area	Percentage
Niche (specialized domain—e.g., medical)	22.41%
KM (knowledge management)	18.97%
BPR (business process related)	12.07%
Sales (sales, marketing, CRM)	12.07%
Tools (e.g., software configuration)	10.34%
PM (project management)	8.62%
HR (human resources)	5.17%
MISC (miscellaneous)	3.45%
PR (public relations/communications)	3.45%
Strategy	3.45%

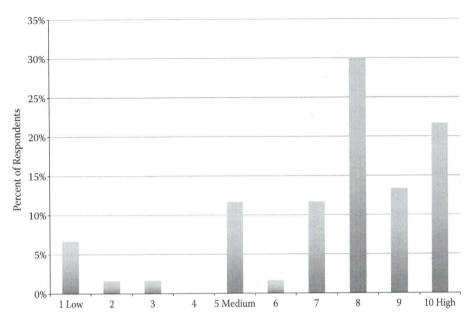

Using a rating scale from Low (1) to High (10), Rate How Strategic Is Your Knowledge with the Mission and Vision of Employer?

Figure 4.5   Most respondents believe that their knowledge is critical at a strategic level affecting the organization's ability to achieve its strategic goals or mission.

Only one in five organizations has a knowledge retention strategy (see Figure 4.6). A high level of knowledge criticality (7.4 average rating) suggests the organization would behave in ways to retain critical knowledge and thus maintain business continuity. In this sample, four of five did not have a retention strategy as part of a succession plan or workforce development activity, but almost two in five stated that a backup expert was present in the organization with their critical knowledge—suggesting that organizations use informal management practices or culture to spread critical knowledge across the organization. Exactly the same proportion was obtained by Monster (2007). Eighty percent of the sample answered no when asked if their organization had a formal knowledge retention strategy.

Formal retention strategies for the 20% that had them described them as:

- Learning as part of business processes
- Cross-training
- Succession planning, process asset knowledge library, shadowing, formal coaching, and mentoring
- Continuous dialogue (daily) on all core issues

- Joint research
- Open-door policy/trusted relationships
- Several instructors identified and employed
- Typical backup and archive of electronic information
- "Turn over" files are developed for specialized applications
- All IT records backed up—all core business functions, proposals, deliverables—filed in associated databases
- Systematic monitoring of experts leaving in the next ten years, formal expert debriefing process

Most respondents never used formal phased retirement programs. Respondents were asked about the frequency with which they used knowledge transfer mechanisms in the organization. Transfer mechanisms were described as being used daily, weekly, monthly, quarterly, sometimes, or never.

The knowledge transfer mechanism almost never used was a formal phased retirement program (86%), followed by the continuity book (58%; see Figure 4.7). Other transfer mechanisms were more uniformly used with deskside reviews, informal knowledge sharing, formal mentoring, and online communities of practice more frequently used. The most frequently used mechanisms for transfer seem to be directed, focused, personal, and intraorganizational (except for communities of practice).

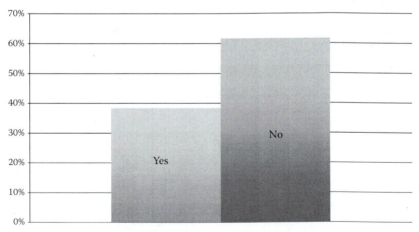

Percentage of Respondents Answering Yes/No About Having a Backup Expert

Figure 4.6 Thirty-eight percent of respondents state they have a backup expert with their critical knowledge, but surprisingly 80% do not believe their firms have a formal retention strategy in place. The result implies that management practices are used to reduce the risk of critical knowledge being concentrated in a single person.

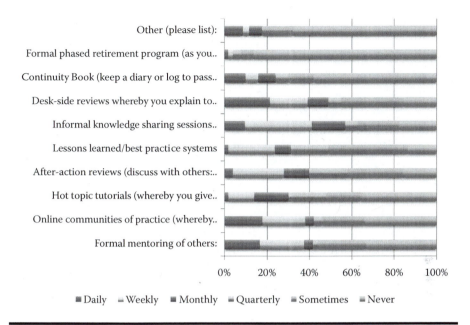

Figure 4.7   How often do you use each of the following methods in your organization? Most respondents use desk-side reviews and informal knowledge sharing methods most frequently.

Many organizations do not have formal knowledge retention strategies (80%), resulting in use of more informal and thus less costly techniques for knowledge transfer. In some cases, such as communities of practice, it is likely that cost is spread across many organizations and professional associations, thus reducing initial investment in technology for any one participant organization. Communities of practice also may allow isolated experts to share experiences and develop each other as eventual backups.

Nature of Work

Knowledge workers have different job profiles: varied research methodologies, processes, tools, transfer mechanisms, and retention constraints. The survey asked participants about the nature of daily or weekly work duties (e.g., routine procedural, judgment-based, etc.), retention of work products, preference for sharing useful information produced by others (e.g., magazine article), and constraints they faced in accessing and sharing, as well as tools or resources they preferred in doing their jobs. Two questions also were designed to explore the expected asymmetry of those needing more sharing but who also were less likely to share.

Respondents were asked to describe frequent job activities (see Figure 4.8). Activity choices were described generically in terms of decision making, problem solving, complexity, independence, skill, and knowledge. For example, answering specific questions from a known source likely requires both lower skill and autonomy than answering when sources are unknown and requires research in addition to answer preparation.

Most responded that their frequent job activities tended to be complex, requiring judgment, self-directed research or general research activity, and preparations of reports or other written communications. The most frequent activity was multi-source data gathering, in which the respondent must find and synthesize information in answering a specific question. This suggests some autonomy and perhaps seniority as respondents are allowed—on a regular basis—more self-direction and exploratory freedom in accomplishing their jobs. Seniority and empowered status of the sample also were implied, as 67% responding said they developed proposals to recommend new programs, projects, procedures, or processes.

The percentages of sample respondents were lowest for step-by-step instructions provided in unwritten form to others (45%) or routine procedures (49%), giving further support to the autonomy given survey respondents in day-to-day job activities.

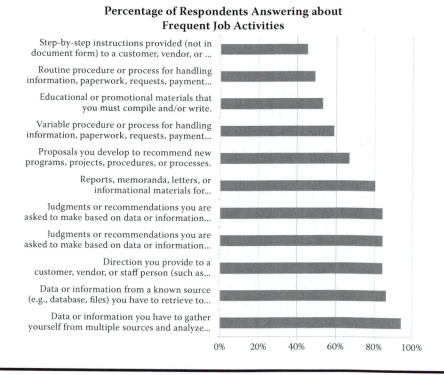

Percentage of Respondents Answering about Frequent Job Activities

Figure 4.8 Respondents generally prepared data by gathering and analyzing it themselves. Most respondents participated in job activities suggesting more independence. Rote job activities were generally the least selected.

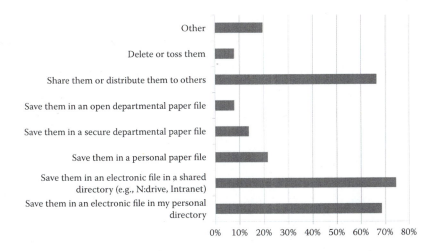

Figure 4.9 Most respondents had stated a preference for saving and sharing a work product. Impediments to sharing were not explored but could include information security policies and regulatory requirements which would impact work product retention practices.

Respondents were asked to describe what they did with work products once the main task was completed (see Figure 4.9). Most had a clear preference for sharing them (more than 60%) and storing them in a shared electronic location (75%) or a personal electronic location (69%). Still, a large number of respondents would delete or toss out the work product, perhaps thinking that the work product was no longer current. Perhaps this represents the view that they should be allowed to "forget" and that blind accumulation is not worthwhile because it stifles innovation. Knowledge does have a shelf life (Scalzo, 2006; Monkey, 2005).

Few respondents had a propensity to share openly available ancillary information, although they would share their own work products. Formal sharing of a completed work product was much more likely than informal sharing of ancillary information. Few of the respondents had a propensity to share due to workplace competition. When asked about sharing information useful to colleagues, just 36% would distribute a copy personally, and only one-fifth would tell colleagues about it (see Figure 4.10). Even fewer would use other modalities to inform colleagues of relevant, open-source information. Our question implied that the information was public (magazine, announcement, etc.).

Low tendency to share may be related to organizational power and influence. There are many interpretations:

■ Knowledge is a competitive advantage, thus sharing could reduce a person's role and visibility in the organization.

- Colleagues are already saturated with information—overloaded—so additional sharing may not be appreciated and might even be interpreted as a distraction.
- Regulations might preclude sharing (e.g., no access to the Internet from work machines, Chinese walls).
- Organizations are so large and effectively compartmentalized into silos that it is difficult to identify appropriate target colleagues.
- Time, budget, and classified security concerns were mentioned as constraints to sharing.

For help in doing their jobs, most respondents preferred electronic documents and people to talk with in real time (see Figure 4.11). Most respondents (more than 70%) viewed electronic forms of documents and a person they could talk to in real time as most preferred forms of help resources to accomplish their jobs. Advice via an online community of practice, Web-based utility, and availability of printed documents were considered helpful by about half the respondents. Least preferred (less than 30%) forms of job help were helpline, AV/multimedia material, and specialized software. Other forms of job help listed by respondents included training (general fields and process specialized), access to higher levels of base research (e.g., industry trends), or access to centralized stores of information.

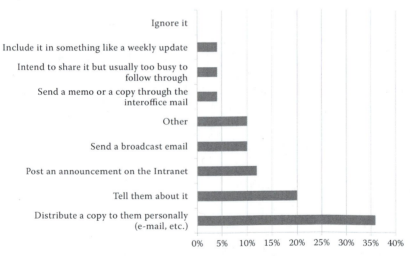

Figure 4.10 Respondents are generally unlikely to share ancillary information. They are much more likely to share a completed work product, with about half as many willing to distribute electronically a helpful piece of information than a finished work product.

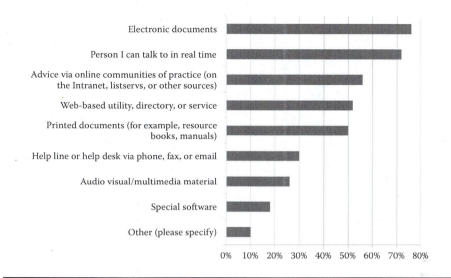

Figure 4.11   **Most respondents would prefer electronic documents and people to talk with in real time in helping them accomplish their job.**

According to respondents, information or knowledge that would improve their job included: training, access to relevant research, development of repositories and cases, well-defined processes, and tools for improving efficiency. Respondents desired a "sense making tool," "prewritten templates to help in proposal writing," and "insight into which vendors were worth recommending over others." Responses generally were related to improved efficiency through better tools, representations, development of repositories, process definitions and documentation, and training.

Respondents confirmed strongly their belief that knowledge-sharing processes and capture templates would help them share knowledge.

General Trends about Facilitating Knowledge Sharing and Tool Availability

Almost 80% of respondents answering the question agreed that they would benefit from processes to help contribute knowledge that is currently undocumented or unshared (see Figure 4.12).

Respondents also believed they could benefit from templates designed to help them capture knowledge more easily, for example, simple Word documents describing elements of a back-to-office report for conference attendance. Seventy-three percent agreed with this.

Sixty-seven percent of respondents would like to have access to introductory materials about a new knowledge domain which they might currently have to acquire from

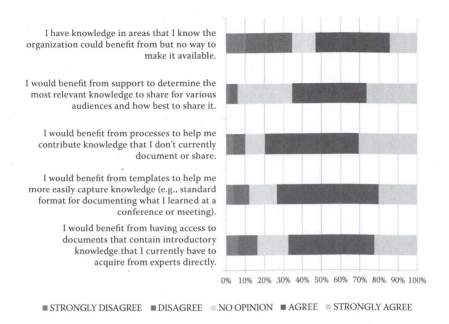

Figure 4.12 Most respondents believe that processes could be defined to help them share knowledge more, and that templates would help capture knowledge more easily. Many also would benefit from access to overview documents to help them get started in a new domain, and that would not then burden experts with basic information requests. Less desirable were the opportunity to benefit from support to help facilitate sharing by determining what and to whom knowledge should be directed. Just over half felt that they had knowledge to contribute to areas important to their organization, but did not have a way to make it less tacit.

experts. At least two dynamics may be evident in that (1) experts act as gatekeepers even for introductory materials in their recognized domain and (2) there is a real desire by requesters not to burden experts with potentially fundamental requests for information.

Sixty-six percent agreed to the potential benefit of having a facilitator to identify relevant knowledge to share and best sharing practices.

The lowest agreement rate was 52% who believed they had knowledge that would be beneficial to their employer but had no mechanism by which to make it available. This could be due to the lack of mechanisms, training in how to codify tacit knowledge, or time budgeted to documentation and codification, and requires more research.

Case Study: IFC, World Bank Group Industry Experts

Forty industry or sector experts in the International Finance Corp. (IFC) were contacted by e-mail and asked to participate in a materially similar survey. Eleven responded and fully participated in the survey, so it is appropriate to treat results as a qualitative case rather than a definitive statistical comparison with the broad sample.

IFC is the private-sector arm of the World Bank Group. It is a not-for-profit organization supporting development through the private sector in emerging and frontier markets. Investments are made on the basis of financial and other criteria (additionality is attained on the basis of IFC's expertise in environment, governance, and social criteria). As a result there is a strong role for experts who specialize in particular industries with deep technical, operational, and financial knowledge.

About half of respondents were working in the Washington headquarters, with the other half in locations around the world. Most respondents were planning to retire within the next ten years (77% IFC versus general survey of 46%), and 91% had been working at IFC between two and ten years, confirming that IFC's industry experts are mid-career hires who tend to stay through early retirement.

Respondents were recognized experts in sectors including private-sector investment in the automotive industry and packaging, general manufacturing, pulp and paper production and management expertise, project evaluation, global trade finance, telecommunications, livestock industry, global benchmarking, global contacts, building materials sector, cement industry, and rural finance. None of the respondents were from KM or related information fields. The nature of their jobs was very specialized, with few working on rote tasks. Most respondents' job activities involved independent, specialized activities around investment and strategy.

In the IFC sample, 44% stated there was a backup expert with their critical knowledge (38% for the general sample). IFC respondents also thought their knowledge was of slightly lower strategic importance (6.9 average versus 7.4 for the general sample). Further reinforcing this assessment was the fact that relatively low-cost techniques, such as mentoring, deskside reviews, and informal sharing, were the most frequently utilized methods of sharing. The culture of sharing was more evident in the IFC sample, with as many as 88% saving work products in shared electronic drives and 75% distributing ancillary materials to colleagues personally via e-mail. The most preferred resource for helping with current job activities was electronic documents (100% response), followed by 63% wanting a person to talk to or Web-based utility or directory.

Respondents agreed that they could make their jobs better by having access to specialized industry resources (e.g., McKinsey global cases database) and less overhead for processing projects, including access to a good CRM system.

Impediments to accessing or sharing knowledge involved access to resources, such as time, overwork, and lack of assistants or apprentices for most respondents.

IFC has set knowledge management as a fundamental strategy pillar and is currently in the process of setting up communities of practice to help with both sharing and retention of knowledge (IFC, 2008b).

As one IFC expert summed it up, "Life is perpetual school, including for experts. The information I'll need tomorrow will be available probably only tomorrow, especially in an extremely fast moving industry like the one I advise for."

Findings and Recommendations

- Respondents primarily work for large U.S. organizations.
- Fewer than 30% plan to leave their present employer or retire within the next five years.
- Most believe their knowledge is highly strategic and critical to the enterprise.
- Eighty percent say their organization has no formal knowledge retention strategy in place, but 38% have a backup expert in the organization.
- Formal phased retirement and continuity book (mechanisms identified for retaining knowledge) were almost never used by respondents. Informal knowledge sharing sessions (storytelling, etc.) and deskside reviews were cited as the most prevalent forms of knowledge transfer.
- Without formal knowledge retention programs, most initiatives are likely organic and fragmented, potentially very small parts of fragmented administrative budgets, or locked up in large IT projects (e.g., document management and workflow systems).
- Respondents recognize the need for retention, capture, and sharing devices, but inevitably small budget allocations to developing a culture of knowledge retention and management will likely continue to hinder an organization's capacity to retain its keepers of critical knowledge or the knowledge itself for use by others who are coached into developing appropriate expertise.

References

De Long, D. (2005). Six mistakes to avoid when implementing an aging workforce strategy, Monograph online, retrieved from http://www.lostknowledge.com/articles-resources/six-mistakes-to-avoid.php.

De Long, D. and Davenport, T. (2003). Better practices for retaining organizational knowledge: Lessons from the leading edge. *Employment Relations Today*, 51–63.

Ebrahimi, M., A. Saives, and W. Holford (2008). Qualified ageing workers in the knowledge management process of high-tech businesses, *Journal of Knowledge Management*, 12, 2, 124–43.

Frigo, M. (2006). Knowledge retention: A guide for utilities, *Journal of the American Water Works Association*, 98, 9, 81–84.

Hesketh, B. (1997). Dilemmas in training for transfer and retention, *Applied Psychology: An International Review*, 46, 4, 317–86.

IFC (2008a). The role of the private sector in health in Africa: Findings and IFC strategy, retrieved from http://www.ifc.org/ifcext/healthinafrica.nsf/AttachmentsByTitle/IFC_Presentation_English/$FILE/IFC_Presentation_English.pdf.

IFC (2008b). IFC management response to IEG-IFC, independent evaluation of IFC's development results 2008: IFC's additionality in supporting private sector development, retrieved from http://www.ifc.org/ifcext/ieg.nsf/AttachmentsByTitle/IEDR2008IFCManagementResponse/$FILE/IEDR2008_IFC+Management+Response.pdf.

Inman, D. and R. Inman (2004). Coping with the impending labor shortage. *Journal of Organizational Culture, Communications and Conflict*, 8, 1.

Kennedy, D. (2006). Attrition rate of mature engineers, *Engineering Management Journal*, 18, 3, 36–40.

Lahti, R. and M. Beyerlein (2000). Knowledge transfer and nanagement consulting: A look at 'the firm,' *Business Horizons*, 65–74.

Lee, T. and S. Maurer (1997). The retention of knowledge workers with the unfolding model of voluntary turnover, *Human Resource Management Review*, 7, 3, 247–75.

Liebowitz, J. (2003). A knowledge management implementation plan at a leading US technical government organization: A case study, *Knowledge and Process Management*, 10, 4, 254–59.

Liebowitz, J. (2008). Knowledge retention survey, retrieved June 10, 2008, from https://www.surveymonkey.com.

Liebowitz, J. (2009). *Knowledge Retention: Strategies and Solutions*. New York: Auerbach Publishing.

Liebowitz, J. and J. Liebowitz (2006). Trends and management challenges of the changing workforce: Knowledge management as a possible remedy, *LabMedicine*, 37, 6, 335–38.

Lintern, G., F. Diedrich, and D. Serfaty (2002). Engineering the community of practice for maintenance of organizational knowledge, Human Factors and Power Plants, IEEE 7th Human Factors Meeting, Scottsdale, Arizona, 6-7–6-13.

Lord, R. and P. Farrington (2006). Age-related differences in the motivation of knowledge workers, *Engineering Management Jounal*, 18, 3, 20–26.

Losey, S. (July 6, 2008). Retirements slowing down, retrieved Aug. 8, 2008, from http://www.federaltimes.com/index.php?S=3612001.

McManus, D., A. Snyder, and L. Wilson. The knowledge management imperative, retrieved Aug. 8, 2008, from http://www.knowledgeharvesting.org/documents/The%20Knowledge%20Management%20Imperative.pdf.

Monkey (2005). Knowledge retention and the importance of forgetting, retrieved Aug. 8, 2008, from http://blog.monkeymagic.net/archives/2005/06/01/knowledge_retention_and_the_importance_of_forgetting.html.

Monster (2007). Organizational knowledge retention report, retrieved Aug. 8, 2008, from http://media.monster.com/a/i/intelligence/pdf/KnowledgeRetentionReport_Summer2007.pdf.

Parise, S., R. Cross, and T. Davenport (2006). Strategies for preventing a knowledge-loss crisis. *MIT Sloan Management Review*, 47, 4, 31–38.

Philip, M. and B. Turnbull (2006). A study into the effectiveness of unqualified GP assistants, *British Journal of Nursing*, 15, 14, 782–86.

Rawstory (Mar. 30, 2007). U.S. government 'outsourcing its brain,' from http://rawstory.com/news/2007/U.S._Government_outsourcing_its_brain_0330.html.

Ray, D. and B. Snyder (2006). Strategies to address the problem of exiting expertise in the electric power industry, Proceedings of the 39th Hawaii International Conference on System Sciences.

Salmon, M., J. Yan, H. Hewitt, and V. Guisinger (2007). Managed migration: The Caribbean approach to addressing nursing services capacity, *Health Services Research*, 42, 3 II, 1354–72.

Scalzo, N. (2006). Memory loss? Corporate knowledge and radical change, *Journal of Business Strategy*, 27, 4, 60–69.

Stillwell, B., K. Diallo, P. Zurn, M. Vujicic, O. Adams, and M. Poz (2004). Migration of health-care workers from developing countries: Strategic approaches to its management, *Bulletin of the World Health Organization*, 82, 8.

Szulanski, G. (1996). Exploring internal stickiness: Impediments to the transfer of best practice within the firm, *Strategic Management Journal*, 17, 27–43.

Wilson, T. (2002). The nonsense of 'knowledge management,' *Information Research*, 8, 1, retrieved from http://informationr.net/ir/8-1/paper144.html.

Wysocki, B. (Mar. 30, 2007). Is U.S. government 'outsourcing its brain'? Boom in tech contracts sparks complex debate; A mecca in Virginia, *The Wall Street Journal*.

KNOWLEDGE MANAGEMENT APPLICATIONS IN PUBLIC HEALTH

Chapter 5

Examples of Knowledge Management in Public Health

Angela M. Fix, Sterling Elliott, and Irene Stephens

Contents

Introduction

Definitions of knowledge management range from the practical to the conceptual and philosophical. The Association of State and Territorial Health Officials (ASTHO) publication *Knowledge Management for Public Health Professionals* provides a broad conceptual framework for better understanding knowledge management and its implications for public health. Fundamentally, knowledge management is the process of organizing and analyzing information to make it understandable and applicable to problem solving or decision making. This basic definition underlies the use of knowledge management by public health organizations.

This chapter provides an overview of practical approaches to knowledge management in public health and represents an update of the 2005 ASTHO publication titled "Examples of Knowledge Management in Public Health Practice." The intent of the 2005 publication was to provide public health officials with basic information about the challenges they may face and the components of knowledge management they need to consider, and to illustrate examples undertaken by other public health agencies. It also provided a list of resources that public health officials could use to explore these components in greater detail. This updated chapter provides an overview of knowledge management from the perspective of state governmental public health and revisits the case studies highlighted in the original publication.

Challenges of Knowledge Management

Most organizations, including public health agencies, face common challenges in attempting to manage knowledge. These include:

Volume of information: Public health agencies manage vast quantities of information, most of which is collected for a specific purpose and not intended for "information reuse." The sheer volume of information managed by most agencies is both a strong incentive as well as an impediment to being able to manage knowledge.

Information security: Public health information is derived from many sources and is frequently considered private or confidential. Though individual datasets may not reveal personal information, combining information from different sources might inadvertently reveal personal information about individuals. Agencies must ensure access controls to maintain information security and confidentiality.

Quality: Ensuring and understanding data quality are critical requirements for knowledge management but difficult to do. Standardized methods for processing data are needed, as is good documentation (or metadata). Data collected for one purpose and integrated with other data or used for another purpose may no longer meet data quality parameters established during initial data collection.

Ability to access and use information: While many agencies collect and compile large volumes of information, few have established the means to access and analyze the data with appropriate tools. This challenge is related to the challenge of maintaining security and the means for users to understand the quality of the data.

Components of Knowledge Management

There are four core components that an organization must consider when attempting to manage its knowledge:

- The governance or leadership that commits to an organizational structure capable of managing knowledge and the subsequent policies that guide the use of the technology.
- The quality and quantity of the data and information that is to be managed (the content).
- The processes, standards, or guidelines that will be used to collect, manage, and disseminate information.
- The technology that supports all of the above.

Many public health agencies are currently developing systems to better understand, manage, and use their existing information, as well as collaborating to create new repositories of knowledge. These activities require commitment and input from all levels and perspectives within the agency. Senior management must provide the leadership to develop a clear understanding of the business needs for knowledge and commit to the changes knowledge management requires. This leadership represents the governance component. Operations staff and content experts can contribute to the process through documentation and organization of the content. Involvement from information technology staff is critical when deploying the technology infrastructure. Technology expertise helps to facilitate knowledge management, but leadership sets the course and drives it through intra-agency policies and large state government policies that set the parameters or use.

Governance

The first step in knowledge management is to understand the business of the agency and how data, information, and knowledge support that business. An agency requires leaders willing to ask difficult questions about what and how work is done. This includes understanding where knowledge exists, how information flows, what data are collected, and who is involved in these processes. This is all part of the "governance" of knowledge management. Organizations must have the ability to critically evaluate information-sharing structures and identify potential bottle-necks. Original mandates of organizations may change, but the organizational structure often remains tailored toward the original mandate. Information silos or stand-alone information systems can often result from this organizational inertia; however, they are more likely the results of siloed and one-time funding streams. In the classic information silo, the focus is inward, and all communication is vertical. Managers in the silo serve as information gatekeepers, making coordination and communication among departments difficult to achieve. Information silos usually exist because:

- There are no perceived benefits or incentives to an individual or division for sharing information.
- There are no established forums where individuals from different divisions can share information.
- The information that is shared in its original collection format may not be meaningful to individuals outside of the collecting office.

Organizations have adopted a variety of strategies to provide governance. States have begun to tackle the issue of information silos among public health and health care sectors by supporting health information exchange efforts. In Minnesota, the Minnesota e-Health Advisory Committee was charged by the state legislature with making recommendations to the commissioner of the Minnesota Department of Health (MDH) on achieving the vision of the Minnesota eHealth Initiative. This vision is to "accelerate the use of health information technology to improve health-care quality, increase patient safety, reduce healthcare costs and enable individuals and communities to make the best possible health decisions." Specifically, the committee advises on efforts to realize state mandates on the adoption of interoperable Electronic Health Records (EHRs), electronic prescribing, and data standards that support interoperability. System interoperability is the technological base for the exchange of information among public health and health care entities. The committee consists of representatives of all relevant stakeholder organizations, from provider organizations, health care facilities, state and local government, health plans, and consumers.

Effective leadership helps set the direction for a knowledge management approach and maintains the impetus for organizational transformation. Senior management can:

- Initiate an information-sharing culture.
- Develop mechanisms that recognize individual efforts to improve the quality of data.
- Create a forum for discussions on information-sharing needs and identify bottlenecks.

- Invest in technology that can make information useful and meaningful to many individuals (e.g., visualization tools).

Minnesota: Minnesota e-Health Initiative

A 2007 statute mandated that all health care providers in Minnesota have interoperable EHR systems by 2015. To reach the 2015 goal, the commissioner of the Minnesota Department of Health, in consultation with the Minnesota e-Health Advisory Committee, is charged with developing a plan to realize this mandate, including the adoption of uniform standards to ensure system interoperability. The stress of the legislation on system interoperability shows the foresight of leadership on ensuring the foundation of an information-sharing culture in the state. For its part, the Minnesota e-Health Advisory Committee is made up of twenty-six leaders representing consumers, the health care delivery community, purchasers, and public health. With its varied membership, the committee represents the broad array of stakeholder interests in state health information technology adoption and use. The committee ensures that the activities around health information exchange and technology adoption occur in a focused, coordinated manner.

Much of the work of the Minnesota e-Health Initiative is carried out in workgroups, which provide a forum for discussion and identification of bottlenecks and obstacles to the vision. Work groups make recommendations to the committee on standards; privacy and security; population health and public health information systems; and communications, education, and collaboration, as well as implementation of the 2015 mandate. Specific tasks have included:

- Developing a statewide plan to ensure that all providers and care-delivery settings have effectively implemented interconnected EHRs by 2015.
- Selecting health-data standards for the exchange of medication histories, prescriptions, and laboratory test results.
- Identifying ways to ensure that the adoption of health information technology leads to improvements in quality and in population health.
- Identifying which public health information systems are most critical to modernize as part of meeting the 2015 mandate and for protecting and improving the public's health.

The ultimate promise of all the e-health activities is that linking health information across entities adds significant meaning and utility to that information for all participants, from government to health care provider to consumers.

Content

Data, information, skills, and expertise can be thought of as the content resources of an organization. Organizations often create content on an ad hoc basis and seldom have procedures to make the information accessible beyond the individuals who collect and manage the information (frequently perceived to be the only users). Making content electronically available does not necessarily ensure that it will be most useful. Data may need to be reformatted, translated, or integrated to optimize use.

Organizations often provide their staff and customers with an organizational view of their content (e.g., structured by hierarchy and divisions). Although this can be useful in understanding how an organization works, it tends to reinforce information silos and discourage the sharing of information. This structure also is not useful to an outsider who is interested in themes that cross the agency structure. Content should be packaged and presented in targeted ways tailored to the user-specific needs and interests. An example of such an approach was implemented by the California Department of Public Health.

Most knowledge management systems deal with explicit knowledge (e.g., tangible knowledge that can be categorized and organized). Tapping into an organization's tacit knowledge—the knowledge held by individuals and their skills and expertise—is challenging. Social networking has been made more accessible through the implementation of systems that attempt to catalog an organization's human capital. By making the catalog available to individuals in an organization, tacit knowledge can be captured and transformed into discrete information that is searchable and can be organized.

California: Targeted Content

The California Department of Public Health recently redesigned its Web site to provide users with specific content based on users' specific needs and interests. The previous site architecture was closely aligned with the structure and hierarchy of the organization, which proved to be confusing and nonintuitive for users outside the agency. The new site architecture focuses on the needs of the general public as well as target audiences, such as public health professionals, clinicians, and students, in the way it presents data and information.

Processes

Formal processes are essential to the creation and management of knowledge repositories. The processes developed need to be responsive to the organization's business needs, as well as able to be implemented within the organizational culture. Individuals within an organization are seldom aware of the complex array of information managed by the agency. Steps to find, understand the quality of, and manage data and information can provide a framework for enhancing agency knowledge.

One of the first steps an organization can take is to inventory existing content. This can be as simple as creating a list of all the repositories of information and intended purposes, as well as how they are currently used. Large organizations with hundreds of knowledge repositories may need to invest more resources to inventory all the databases that exist. One strategy is to create a metadata system that allows knowledge owners to add information about their knowledge repositories and allows others in the organization to search and locate the repositories. Another strategy that an organization can use to locate content is to organize knowledge resources by cataloging the repositories into discreet areas that are agreed upon and understood by stakeholders. This can be achieved by developing a common vocabulary, which allows information to be organized into identifiable categories.

The processes of inventorying and cataloging data are essential. This is especially true for the public health sector, where there is a need to share information vertically within an organization and horizontally among organizations.

Technology

Technology plays a major role in organizations responsible for managing large volumes of electronic information. There are many different technologies that can assist in a knowledge management approach, including data warehouses, geographic information systems, electronic dashboards, document management systems, visualization tools, and query and search utilities.

Organizations often pursue a technical solution without addressing the processes and governance structure that will be needed to make the content useful. Organizations can overcome this potential pitfall by working to first review their governance and business practices and then adapt them to make the best use of a technology solution instead of trying to force current business practices to meet the specifications of the technology.

Technology solutions also tend to be purchased on an ad hoc basis to solve specific problems. This leads to the deployment of multiple systems, which often are not compatible with each other. Some organizations, such as the Wisconsin Department of Health, are addressing this problem by adopting an enterprise architecture approach to technology and organizing their technological infrastructure by business practices and activities.

The volume and complexity of information in the public health field are increasing, making it difficult for agencies and individuals to keep track of all the information necessary to conduct their business. Increased collaboration between public health agencies and other organizations involved in complementary and supplementary fields has fueled the need to take a knowledge management approach that can organize and integrate information and present it in multiple formats. The Kentucky Department of Public Health benefited from university researchers using a community-based method to gather information on knowledge management, which later led to the development of one of the state's regional health information organizations.

Wisconsin: Enterprise Architecture

For more than two years, the Wisconsin Department of Health & Family Services has been running the SAS Business Intelligence System to bring together information from multiple systems and present a consolidated view of the data. The department created an enterprise knowledge management system by integrating detection, monitoring, analysis, and response systems. The SAS Business Intelligence Server gives the department the ability to access virtually any data source and combine multiple data sources and platforms in a single query.

The system has grown and increased in use to support analysis, visualization, and reporting (AVR) for several public health programs. The department is considering expanding the requirements to include electronic medical record data exchange with public health systems. Wisconsin public health leadership is working toward an information-sharing culture by developing a strategic planning exercise for the Public Health Information Network (PHIN) AVR service (i.e., SAS Business Intelligence System and ESRI ArcGIS Server), which was to be completed by late 2009. Staff also is creating views for the PHIN AVR Web portal to enable automated reporting to produce PDF reports, create data tools for state and local public health departments, and analytic tools for epidemiologists.

Kentucky: Louisville Health Information Exchange (LouHIE)

Several years ago, the Kentucky Department of Public Health and researchers from the University of Louisville sought to develop an electronic dashboard called *VisPlex* (Visualization Complexity) to summarize large quantities of information graphically as part of its bioterrorism preparedness efforts. Cross-organization is critical to homeland security efforts, and the department sought to address the need to present complex data from multiple agencies in a concise manner. The purpose of *VisPlex* was to provide a visual interface to large volumes of data and provide decision makers with the level of detail needed to make informed decisions. While this project is no longer operational, the research behind *VisPlex* provided the foundation for the Louisville Health Information Exchange, or LouHIE.

LouHIE became a nonprofit corporation in January 2006, and was developed to improve quality and decision support in the health care community for consumers and providers. This HIE is not yet functional, but involves stakeholders from public health, academia, medical and insurance providers, governmental agencies, employers, and consumer groups. Funding from Medicaid Transformation Grants has given rise to the initial business model, and vendors are still being sought to develop the system. An independent board of directors was formed to further develop the organization, while its governance and committee structure was shaped around earlier research efforts at the university. Patients in metropolitan Louisville will have the option to open an electronic health record account, which allows authorized health care providers and pharmacies access to medical data via a master patient index at the state level. In addition, LouHIE is supported by the Kentucky eHealth Network.

Conclusion

As is evident from the range of examples, knowledge management includes a diverse array of activities within the field of public health. Many organizations are attempting to bring order to their often chaotic and difficult-to-use collections of data. When the components of knowledge management—governance, content, process, and technology—are identified and addressed, organizations can begin to set a course that creates a significant asset from scattered, siloed stores of information. This asset, in the form of managed knowledge, contributes to a learning organization and more effective and efficient business practices.

Knowledge Management Resources

Knowledge management for public health officials, available by request, e-mail: publications@astho.org.

The Journal of Knowledge Management, available online at http://info.emeraldinsight.com/products/journals/journals.htm?id=jkm.

U.S. government knowledge management Web site, http://www.km.gov, accessed July 12, 2005.

Association of State and Territorial Health Officials (2004). Data sharing with covered entities under the HIPAA privacy rule: A review of three state public health approaches, available by request, e-mail: publications@astho.org.

Doctor, J. (2003). Knowledge management best practices for service and support, ServiceWare Technologies white papers, available online at http://whitepapers.techrepublic.com.

Naidoo, D. (2002). Organisational culture and subculture influences on the implementation and outcomes of aspects of internal quality assurance initiatives, Technikon Northern Gauteng, available from http://www.ecu.edu.au/conferences/herdsa/main/papers/non-ref/pdf/DNaidoo.pdf, accessed July 12, 2005.

TFPL (2004). Knowledge management skills map, available from http://www.tfpl.com/assets/applets/km_skillsmap_2000.pdf, accessed July 12, 2005.

Tobin, T. (2003). Ten principles for knowledge management success, ServiceWare Technologies white paper, available online at http://whitepapers.techrepublic.com.

Acknowledgments

Minnesota: The Minnesota e-Health Initiative
 Martin LaVenture, PhD, MPH
 Director, Public Health Informatics
 Minnesota Department of Health

California: Targeted Content
 Gwendolyn Doebbert, MA, MS
 Strategic Planning Project Manager
 Chief, Strategic Health Information Policy & Planning
 California Department of Public Health

Wisconsin: Enterprise Architecture
 Lawrence P. Hanrahan, PhD, MS
 Director of Public Health Informatics
 Chief Epidemiologist
 Wisconsin Department of Health Services

Kentucky: Louisville Health Information Exchange (LouHIE)
 Judah Thornewill
 Director, Collaborative Community Research
 Department of Health Management and Systems Sciences
 University of Louisville School of Public Health and
 Information Sciences

 April Smith, PMP
 eHealth Project Manager
 Office of Information Technology
 Kentucky Cabinet for Health and Family Services

Chapter 6

Building Knowledge Management in an International Health NGO

Richard Iams and Patricia Ringers

Contents

Embarking on Knowledge Management

Specific criteria must be defined and evaluated prior to the initiation and implementation of any knowledge management (KM) system. These criteria will differ among various organizations but may be assessed with four basic questions: What is knowledge management? Why do we want it? How do we get it? What do we do with it? It is especially critical that each of these areas be fully appraised prior to engaging human and fiscal capital in an enterprise for which there may be limited or competing resources. In this manner, a fully informed decision weighing available resources, level of commitment, and cultural preparedness for a knowledge management system—including both process and technology support—may be made. This case study reviews these issues as they emerged within one public health organization.

Background

JHPIEGO, founded in 1973, was developed as the Johns Hopkins Program in International Education for Gynecology and Obstetrics. Building on expertise in family planning and reproductive health issues facing low-resource countries, the organization has evolved to include training and health delivery systems in maternal and child health, HIV, and other related public health initiatives affecting women and families. As an organization rooted in providing direct educational and experiential learning through a vast array of trainers, personal exchanges are of the utmost value. The majority of U.S.-based JHPIEGO staff spend time traveling to these countries and working with local staff. "Face time" is an essential cultural concept. The social networks created have contributed to JHPIEGO's long-standing presence in areas needing assistance with critical public health issues. While e-mail has become a necessary tool for business communication, meetings and personal interactions are important tools for staff to connect and share knowledge, experiences, and solutions with one another. Although the use of information and telecommunication technologies continues to grow in low-resource settings, direct and personal connections remain an important factor in building credibility and achieving public health results.

JHPIEGO promotes the use of evidenced-based practices to demonstrate effectiveness and sustainability. These practices are tested, monitored, and evaluated to demonstrate results and assess desired impact. However, these practices are not always as replicable in the same manner as other business sectors, such as in the manufacturing industry, where standard tools and techniques can be transferred from one controlled operating environment to another, as evidenced by assembly plant relocations. Public health solutions involve great variability, with confounding factors that can impede reproduction of successful activities—or worse, repeating activities that do not produce effective results. These solutions may be impacted by cultural perspectives, in-country political factors, funding budgets and priorities, regional differences in availability of supplies, and availability of knowledgeable people—both administrative and policy experts, as well as clinical/technical experts. As such, the continual exchange of experience, learning, and knowledge is required to be successful. Building on proven techniques, JHPIEGO's experts build upon evidenced-based practices but must often adapt a solution methodology to fit a specific need and environment. Otherwise, limited resources may be utilized in vain to solve local public health issues.

What Is Knowledge Management?

Knowledge management encompasses a range of processes and techniques designed to maximize an organization's intellectual assets. Knowledge management activities are designed to facilitate the collection and sharing of information, promoting reuse, adaptation, and creation of new knowledge. Providing timely and relevant information to the appropriate audience is an important goal and is frequently referenced in value and mission statements for KM efforts. Solutions can be technology-driven, as are the portal applications commonly found in corporate environments or those that promote sharing in a public Internet, social networking environment. They also may be programs designed to capture the experience of tenured staff and domain experts for transfer and exchange with more recent staff and mentees where technology plays a supporting role. Expected results from KM activities may yield an easier, more effective means for employees to find business information needed to conduct their work—relevant and useful results when searching the corporate portal. Or, staff may engage in rich knowledge exchange activities, not necessarily bound by physical proximity or department assignments, which lead to innovative solutions and improved results in business activities.

Challenges Materialized: What Is KM for JHPIEGO?

In many organizations, KM begins as a new or updated initiative to collect, organize, and share the files and information necessary for conducting business, and to improve the findability of relevant information when it is needed by its staff. For JHPIEGO, that means easy access to standardized training manuals, evidenced-based guidelines, program reports, and other information necessary to support its programs. These artifacts document the institutional history of JHPIEGO and the evolution of its best practices. KM also includes the transferring and exchange of expertise between headquarters-based staff and those located in the field as practices are developed, tested, and documented. In addition, KM for JHPIEGO includes a learning component, since understanding and competency of key organizational concepts is important to program implementation. Early KM efforts focused on building online data applications to store key reports and program artifacts as they were created so they could be retrieved later by other staff members. The artifacts typically would be reusable and adaptable, or document program activities for historical record. Additionally, planned and informal activities designed to share the latest practices and innovations provided learning opportunities for staff.

JHPIEGO depends on reliable Web technologies for both external and internal information storage and dissemination to information seekers, as do most organizations. The support tools to create and maintain Web sites are mature and robust. Other typical methods to share information throughout JHPIEGO include: e-mail to broadcast attachments; distribution lists and staff lists designating department assignments; and meetings, reports, minutes, and presentations posted on the intranet. However, these techniques each have drawbacks for achieving maximum KM. The impact of staff meetings and the opportunity to connect with colleagues is limited to attending staff. For JHPIEGO, an organization with more personnel located oversees than at its headquarters, the impact of discussing overall themes addressed in such a meeting has limited reach. Staff lists merely providing phone numbers and departments convey little information about personal expertise and current focus of work. Distribution of meeting minutes via e-mail serves as a perfunctory administrative activity that transfers little knowledge to readers and may seem more like spamming one's own employees. With field staff relying on dial-up Internet connections and reduced connection speeds, Internet time is more effective for conducting work directly related to immediate tasks and communication directly with closest co-workers. Also, there existed many different databases, network file shares, and sources of information which hindered the ability to find in one place related information on a particular subject or activity.

Given these parameters, the internal solutions to creating a KM system could include the use of portal and collaborative tools to save and share programmatic information within project teams and interest areas, decentralize ownership responsibilities for the most current and relevant information to domain experts, and provide means to highlight or notify users of new content availability. These tools could improve information accessibility and availability while staff travel or work offline and offer staff choices as to when and how to access specific information. Other challenges were to reduce the dependence on e-mail, a reliable communication tool, as a file-share method and on network drives to save key files. Access to these network drives while not sitting within the walls of the corporate office could be difficult using standard network security protocols, which were problematic for many working in the field. While e-mail is a reliable message delivery system, use as an organization-wide file-share mechanism can present issues for colleagues with slow and comparatively expensive Internet connections. The portal solutions demonstrate some of the additional capabilities that KM technology can provide beyond traditional e-mail or network shares in supporting everyday activities.

While the current KM system is limited in its scope of reaching all necessary staff, how the culture of JHPIEGO may or may not be supportive of the implementation of a KM system must also be examined. There exists an intrinsic nature within those professionals who seek personal connections and have the desire to solve public health issues at organizations such as JHPIEGO. These organizations reinforce the face-to-face nature of knowledge exchange. It is insufficient to address public health issues solely through expertise gained by academic review and training. Target issues and populations must be understood by first-person experience and involved in the solution-building process for there to be sustainable and successful outcomes. For international public health programs, success is dependent upon social connections and networking, as well as the strength of the underlying evidenced-based practices. As such, the implementation of a KM system which focuses reliance more on the use of computerized systems to retrieve documented knowledge and strategies without supporting personal interactions may be quite challenging.

For the staff at JHPIEGO, conceptual design of a KM system proved to be a challenge. Many staff primarily conceptualized a centrally maintained library of reading materials and documents that they could access by browsing familiar topics or performing a text search. The concept of using a computerized system other than e-mail or a database as a vehicle to independently share personal knowledge and concepts with others, or for online collaboration, was not universally recognized. The ability of such a system to support and enhance current socially dependent practices to improve value to staff also may have been underappreciated.

Why Do We Want It?

KM is desirable for several reasons. Some business sectors depend on an available workforce and technology support that increases volume, output, and efficiencies and can be achieved through strong technology integration among its business processes to help drive growth and support success. However, organizations such as JHPIEGO depend on the knowledge and expertise of their people to continually create new solutions, analyze data, and produce successful results. The pool of trained experts required to support this work may be limited, due to demand in a particular public health area or clinical expertise, country work experience, or language fluency. While some organizations working in commoditized industries can respond to consumer or product demand quickly with potentially less experienced workers, knowledge-based organizations—those that depend on their human capital—rely on workers who can be cross-trained or quickly apply new information to their own specialized experiences.

Each business has its unique ways of getting business done, regardless of how common its domain. Therefore, it is important for organizations to quickly and effectively orient staff to learn their core activities, both administrative and functional. The implementation and utilization of a KM system allow staff to adapt more quickly and expeditiously to changes in operating conditions, new policy guidelines, or directives both internally and externally. A well-designed system should intuitively reflect an organization's strategic activities and areas of focus so all staff, new and tenured, understand current and future priorities.

An effective system allows staff to easily contribute information themselves, to intuitively find information submitted by others, to discover colleagues with related interests, and make connections to build new, collaborative partnerships within the organization. It is important to be able to share recent news, results, and successes publicly in a system that allows this to be found later when it is needed by others. In this manner, new partnerships can be sought with peers at appropriate times, and successes can be celebrated at milestone dates. Awareness of a breadth of activities and opportunities can lead to stronger, more effective programs and service delivery. Programs staffed by informed and connected people may have a higher survival and success rate through the increased ability to share or utilize scarce resources. This transfer of knowledge among experts and public health practitioners is necessary for the sustainability of an organization.

Challenges Materialized: Why Does JHPIEGO Want It?

There is a continual need for experienced public health workers to staff and support ongoing and emergent issues affecting low-resource settings. Many areas facing severe and unexpected public health crises see greater demand for service and care than the existing infrastructure can support. Clinical staff is in short supply, and many people living in rural areas lack convenient access to adequate facilities and trained experts. More critically, the HIV/AIDS crisis, as an example, affects not only the general population but also results in increased morbidity and mortality among those people who have been trained previously to respond to the crisis. As such, there is a great need for the transfer of both knowledge and experience and the ability to tap into existing resources. While some required knowledge is didactic in nature and can be learned independently, other success factors and tacit knowledge are better exchanged by familiar social techniques. A successful KM program must support both explicit and tacit knowledge capture to maximize the value and benefit to the entire organization and increase the reach of its expertise to all audiences.

Other factors lead to the desire for KM as well. Low-resource settings experience "brain drain," where medical students train outside their home country and stay away for a longer duration. While some may return following their training, either immediately or some time thereafter to practice locally, others relocate altogether and are no longer a viable resource for the home community. Few of the countries with the greatest public health needs likely have the resources or capacity to continually reinvest in the formal education required to maintain a sufficient talent pool to combat the brain drain. In other regions, cultural and political circumstances are such that educational opportunities are limited by gender, class, or ethnic status, further limiting the pool of human capital available to meet the latest challenges.

Organizations operating in a variety of public health contexts rely on their human capacity to strategize given a range of domains, from medical research, policy, epidemiology, and anthropology to anticipate and devise response strategies and programs to meet diverse community needs. Advances in practices and techniques, particularly with regard to efforts combating HIV/AIDS, require staff to understand the latest medical standards and to be able to integrate changes into training and service delivery activities in order to continually produce improved public health results for targeted populations. The primary benefactors of successful KM in this arena are those populations with acute public health challenges which organizations such as JHPIEGO seek to mitigate and solve. However, there are many points in between where learning, training, and experience must be shared to ensure timely and effective use of limited resources.

Internally, organizations must ensure that staff is trained and aware of existing expertise. Staff that possess or have ready access to knowledge and skills complementary to their own may offer more value to their customer. They can provide a better solution than initially requested. Awareness of other organizational domains provides more opportunities to market and earn additional business. While public health organizations have different missions than commercial companies, the fact remains that they are in competition for limited funds. Offering the most skill and expertise for the same funding as a competitor is an advantage for winning awards and providing continuity of service. Once established, these relationships are important to meeting local public health demands. An appropriately conceptualized and devised KM system could be an invaluable asset for any public health NGO.

For JHPIEGO, the increasing pressure to deliver its high-quality services in shorter time frames with dispersed staff requires new means to connect its experts, who may not have the time availability or travel budget to provide their services directly onsite. Usage of the early file repositories diminished as field staff's access to them remained difficult, news staff's of them was lost, and reliability of e-mail for group communication and file sharing became the norm. In addition, the rise in popularity of instant messaging and PC-based telephony applications provided new, relatively reliable, and generally inexpensive options to have synchronous communications with colleagues. These tools are excellent means for connecting people and are a natural fit for a social organization. Their role in a KM system serves to provide an alternative, and sometimes faster, response to e-mail. However, like e-mail, the exchanges via these communication modes are not easily captured—for the purpose of sharing, learning, and dissemination—and the challenge remains for experts to synthesize and distill important conclusions and concepts for other interested staff.

Early KM efforts focused on using dedicated central staff to collect, store, and be responsible for key material, much like a library functions. Success depended on its "librarians," whether they were technology-centric staff or not, to gather and maintain collections of material created by experts. Yet, these collected files represented a fraction of the total content produced by staff. Versions adapted for a particular program might not be resubmitted to the shared repository collection and instead remain on local computers or on a network file share. It was and continues to be important for JHPIEGO staff to easily locate key materials and findings for which much work evolves. Internally, staff need to share information on program activities and results with those working on similar projects, different teams, or locations. Rather than recreating original material which supported either technical or administrative efforts, materials could be made available so that staff could reuse and adapt them as much as possible, thereby creating more efficient processes and improved work product. Creating a program and system that shifts content ownership closer to the expert is more consistent with efforts to place decision making closer to the field-based programs. This offers the local experts more visibility in the knowledge-sharing process and promotes more awareness across the organization about local interests, activities, and priorities. This introduces additional challenges, as staff would require additional administrative and technology training to achieve competency and proficiency. With limited training budgets, a well-planned and coordinated user support process would need development.

One of the challenges with this approach is the identification and acknowledgment of authorship. As files are altered and adapted, original authorship becomes rather fuzzy. Since many staff working with the organization have academic appointments, and are therefore concerned about authorship, there may be reservations by some to place their efforts in a venue for others to adapt and alter at will. Alternatively, some may be reluctant to post their own work out of the belief they do not have the same level of expertise as other contributors. Thus, much work remains findable through primary contact with those working on a project. Seeking this information by means of a library, which holds useful institutional content, may not be the most effective method for connecting with peers to solve important public health issues.

How Do We Get It?

A KM program begins with recognizing the need and value offered by effecting collection, sharing, and dissemination of the expertise held by its people. Identifying and supporting high-value activities with easy-to-use applications can improve the cycle for knowledge collection, sharing, and using. This should be evident in the first official activity between an organization and a new employee—their first day of work. The decision to hire an individual inherently suggests that an organization recognizes the value and expertise the new hire brings. Using the new employee experience as an example, organizations should devise a roadmap that encompasses those processes and knowledge domain areas that will quickly orient the new employee to key subject matter and experts, while also introducing the new employee, and their own expertise, to relevant divisions of the organization. Organizations should create processes, or enhance those already present, that both inform the new hire—as well as more tenured staff—and connect activities and people within the organization to leverage technology in an effort to capture the output of the social connections and extend them to peers. Organizing the knowledge documented and supported by its people, and making those people easy to reach in an intuitive manner, is an important foundation for building KM.

Challenges Materialized: How Did JHPIEGO Seek KM?

KM was not a program within JHPIEGO as much as it was an area of expertise. Leading and best-practice organizations identify KM executive champions, program leaders, budgets, and other forms of traditional institutional support to effect positive change. However, this support typically requires central and shared funding that similarly provides for other organization-wide efforts led by administrative departments, such as finance, human resources, and information technology. The shared model helps provide for universal support rather than create an imbalance of support—i.e., disparities among programs that have different levels of funding and flexibility to pay for services. In the case of JHPIEGO, many experts in various disciplines are advisers, including KM, and typically provide consultative services to contracted activities executed as programs and projects over a period of time. These may include public health clinical skills and training activities designed to transfer knowledge to practitioners in low-resource settings, for which JHPIEGO has established, evidenced-based practices. The activities also might relate to creating new service delivery programs that must eventually be run and owned by the receiving in-country public health program. Thus, the role of a KM adviser may be to engage with the program team to offer additional or innovative ways to increase the reach of the primary activity by which it is being measured, capture the results for the benefit of others, and support the internal learning of staff by connecting them to these experts. The KM aspect of these funded activities is mostly a supporting activity to ensure that the results are shared among the community of practitioners and peer NGO organizations.

JHPIEGO, like many other organizations working under institutional and government support, is often limited in the administrative funding available to grow KM. While it is necessarily important and beneficial to direct as much funding as possible to the experts and recipients of services, support for KM should be seen as a reinvestment in people and the organization. The long-term results in leading KM organizations are that staff are able to find, use, and adapt existing information most effectively regardless of its form. Files can be located, and experts are accessible. These results provide a return on funding support through better service delivery and an organization prepared to quickly meet the next or unforeseen challenge. These returns are difficult to measure accurately, yet the reports available that cite the amount of time knowledge workers spend seeking information allow the inference that even conservative gains in KM behaviors and effectiveness produce positive results.

Having identified some of the key challenges around people and processes, attempting to create and build a computerized system which captures the experience and knowledge of staff is quite challenging. As the World Bank and USAID became aware of the positive impact of KM systems, more public health programs sought to hire individuals who could build such a system. Unfortunately, KM experts cannot build a KM system for any organization without a tremendous level of input and support from staff. An important role of the KM expert is to facilitate the discussion, debates, and finalization of the strategies that will be used to construct the KM system. Public health leaders who have limited resources need to be aware that in order to establish and maintain a KM system, there needs to be a substantial level of commitment—both time and resources—from the staff. Staff needs to identify, buy in, and promote any solution. A KM system requires an investment of resources. There are various options to minimize technology expenses, though a minimum level of commitment is required to effectively reach all target audiences. More importantly, an organization-wide expectation for all staff to build, grow, and maintain the KM program is vital. In some instances, new staff may need to be hired in order to fill critical support roles. In other cases staff may already be performing KM-related activities; however, the activities may need to be adapted or redirected for better performance and results. In effect, organizations must be willing to support a measure of change.

JHPIEGO's path to KM followed that of many of its peers in public health, as well as organizations outside of the sector, with the goal to more easily support internal sharing and to decentralize content management. Microsoft SharePoint was selected to be a new technology platform for JHPIEGO, which was already standardized on Microsoft software for business office applications. Out-of-the-box features of the new platform offered the ability to provide alternatives to using e-mail and central dependency entirely on technologist support roles to share and disseminate information among global staff. This application could simplify the saving, updating, and retrieval of key domain information and shared operational information with point-and-click features. The domain experts could have a more direct role in sharing relevant information without knowing computer programming code for intranet/Internet publication.

Supporting collaboration and sharing outside the corporate network was another important path for knowledge management. JHPIEGO used the Implementing Best Practices (IBP) Knowledge Gateway—a custom-developed communication tool created within the framework of a consortium of internal public health cooperating agencies. The need to share and collaborate with experts and other parties outside of the corporate network was critical to exchanging knowledge and ideas globally. The IBP Knowledge Gateway was collaborative, like SharePoint and other enterprise-based tools, yet was not limited by corporate security and internal administrative support. It operates in the Internet "cloud" and allowed any member to participate either directly online or via e-mail, regardless of their affiliation. Files could be posted and asynchronous discussions held, either using a Web browser online or via e-mail messages. All interactions could be archived and activity sent as a digest to members. This tool facilitated global participation and knowledge exchange at the lowest technology common dominator, e-mail, while preserving an online record for later discovery. For JHPIEGO, this provided an additional tool to extend the reach of its efforts to train and promote competency of learning in important practices among public health practitioners.

In addition, other technologies were explored to support established techniques and practices in order to improve the sharing and exchange of knowledge. PowerPoint slides are ubiquitous for supporting presentation summaries of technical papers, but only the attendees receive the richest presentations. While bullet points and graphs provide useful information to readers, the story and context offered by the presenter often provide the most compelling call to action. In addition, the collaborative discussion that often ensues during a presentation rarely reaches the offline reader. In response to this, audio recording equipment, used infrequently and installed in a conference room, was piloted for use in recording an internal speaker series. These presentations were recorded and converted for playback from the corporate portal so that field-based and absent staff could listen to presentations at a time convenient for them. This technique was extended to record guest experts so that the rich exchange of ideas could be shared. To further the reach and ease of use of these presentations, third-party software, Articulate Presenter, was used to combine and convert the audio and slides into a standard Internet format that is playback friendly to low-bandwidth Internet connections.

What Do We Do with It?

Once an organization has the foundations for KM in place, it is positioned to maximize the intellectual power and experience of its people and history for innovation. This should result in improved and more effective sharing of knowledge and experiences among peers. Once established, learning through guided processes and self-discovery should be achievable, rather than repeating a means of information warehousing typical of many intranet solutions. Experts, learners, knowledge seekers, and practitioners can be more easily connected using data automatically tracked by the technology. Information useful for knowledge discovery, such as who contributed content and when it was submitted, can be found easily to identify experts and communities of interest beyond staff's daily communication channels. Examining usage can support decision making about processes to support and enhance in order to improve value to users and the organization.

Challenges Materialized: What Does JHPIEGO Do with a KM System?

A system for knowledge management supports discovery and exchange of information and ideas. Building upon existing activities and organizational values, a KM system promotes the sharing of best practices and improved impact of business activities. However, examining the patterns and volume of contributions may identify new teams or concepts where innovations are developing or require additional expertise to flourish. JHPIEGO may collect data that identifies information frequently requested or expertise consulted.

Possessing this data allows for critical analysis to determine where gaps in critical knowledge exist in the KM system. When users cannot retrieve information from a knowledge base as expected, it may suggest that the information can or should exist yet still resides offline on a local hard drive. It also may suggest that knowledge hoarding is occurring and new incentives for sharing need consideration, or more simply that not enough administrative time has been allocated to the capture and contribution process. When combined with human resource staffing information and business activity projections, JHPIEGO may assess where it needs to direct and supplement additional resources. Decisions can be made regarding the availability of experts to staff upcoming projects and support resources necessary to update and adapt expert content.

Metrics were not widely collected to quantitatively measure impacts. KM efforts relied on supporting core activities using best practices to fit the program requirements. So, impact was based more on qualitative and subjective factors. In the case of offering an online learning forum on a public health topic, the basic principles of distance education were applied. However, KM best practices for supporting online communities were offered to support the building of a network of experts rather than merely anonymous attendees in an online course. The distance education component of the forum would determine how well the participants mastered the material. At best, KM impact could have been measured through participant satisfaction or new contacts made as a result of participation. Determining longer-term programmatic impact had yet to be allocated into specific program activity budgets.

Obstacles to Overcome

The need to research ideas, understand buzzwords, and the ability to commit necessary resources before taking on any new project are important for any initiative. KM is not for the weak of heart or the poor of resource. It is challenging by the very nature of its focus: improving the exchange of information and ideas among the people and processes of an organization and using new tools to effect improvements. This can be far more complex than automating tangible and defined procedures for exchanging data forms between offices to complete a typical business transaction.

People will be expected to modify some individual practices and behaviors for the organization to maximize its investment in KM. Continual communication and executive sponsorship is vital.

As with any effort that has the potential to impact everyone, organizations should determine the strategic focus of their KM efforts and determine a roadmap for success. For smaller organizations and those with limited funding to support KM, it may be beneficial to consolidate various roles and duties and identify critical areas. KM may support portals, promote collaboration, artifact collection and preservation, and learning and performance support. However, each activity requires sufficient planning and support to implement and build sustainability. Organizations that successfully implement KM do so in a manner that embeds the principles and practices into daily work so that they grow with the organization and outlast discrete tasks. Technical, financial, and operational practices are not newly created for every time-limited program and work task. Instead, established activities are implemented and adapted into each new program based on unique requirements.

When the appropriate technology platform is selected, testing and gaining user acceptance should not be overlooked. The complete replacement of one system with another system risks alienation and user rejection by key people in the organization. Sufficient time should be budgeted to complete this analysis, and a cross-section of users given defined, sanctioned, and budgeted time to contribute ideas and feedback. Otherwise, a phased implementation may be preferred for organizations such as JHPIEGO, where the primary team responsible is small and has other responsibilities beyond the KM project. While the overall project may take longer to implement, starting small and adding features according to an implementation roadmap that adds user value may provide two benefits. One, it allows a sense that progress is continual as features are added, keeping the solution dynamic and growing. It also allows discovery of issues along the way that impact a small group of early adopting users. These early adopters typically see the long-term advantages of the new solution and frequently are more forgiving and more patient in working through issues. In the case of JHPIEGO, and particularly for its satellite offices and traveling staff, the SharePoint solution suffered from poor performance using low-bandwidth Internet connections, and there was no remedy. While staff located in headquarters, homes with high-speed Internet connections, or field offices with reliable dedicated connections could use the platform to access and share information, those using slower connections were unable to experience the same benefits.

In contrast, use of the IBP Knowledge Gateway in JHPIEGO grew slowly and more through word of mouth. As members of the IBP Consortium—a collaborative of peer organizations working in similar countries and in similar public health topics—JHPIEGO participated and promoted using the Knowledge Gateway for sharing information about consortium business for its technical public health interests, and for collaboration and knowledge sharing. One immediate benefit was that the tool was neutral from corporate bounds, i.e., it did not rely on network security and IT standards by any one organization. Using this custom-developed platform allowed for a better understanding of its strengths and weaknesses before committing to broader use. At the appropriate time, program staff within JHPIEGO identified a task where this platform would support an online forum designed to disseminate the latest public health information on a current topic of interest. Furthermore, this solution had allocated staff to support users and provide new features in response to feedback.

Throughout this online community forum, experts from many countries were engaged in information exchange and new people-to-people connections made in manner and reach not possible, without the travel costs, had JHPIEGO conducted an in-country training. While a report could have been issued more broadly via e-mail and posting on a Web site, it would be difficult to assess true reach of the information, measure how many read the report, or, more importantly, how many understood the information to the degree they could internalize and apply it to their work. Participants in the collaborative forum could exchange ideas and questions, thereby extending the value of the baseline information by contributing their experiences and enriching the entire forum. Since the forum is online, all the material and online dialog is available to review and improvement or expansion by subsequent readers who find it. With this experience, the JHPIEGO team was able to identify and internally market its planning process and platform to other staff needing to share information in a similar environment and with similar requirements. Since the forum's capabilities and value were recognized by program managers, the tool was selected and used by motivated early adopters willing to invest the time to ensure achievement of positive results and impact.

Ownership and role of KM within the organizational structure should be carefully considered. Left as an "a la carte" service, programs and departments can inhibit institutionalization of key KM activities and goals. Staffing and resourcing should allow core services to be provided across the organization so that essential value and user needs are met. At the same time, innovations should be explored and introduced to the organization, as they are shown to produce positive impact.

Furthermore, clear expectations and roles between KM process and technology implementation should be defined. When an imbalance between KM service delivery and technology support decisions occurs, efforts may stall from vague and ambiguous leadership on strategy and roadmapping responsibilities. A standing, interdisciplinary team chartered with growing KM as a program may mitigate conflicts often experienced between KM and IT functions. To achieve a successful KM system in any organization, a well-conceived and effective strategy which accounts for available resources, constraints, and corporate culture must be developed and supported.

Chapter 7

Trying to Revive an Anemic System

A Case Study from USAID's Nutrition Division

Laura Birx

Content

USAID Background

Since 1961, the U.S. Agency for International Development (USAID) has been the principal U.S. agency providing assistance to countries recovering from disaster, trying to escape poverty, and engaging in democratic reforms. USAID provides assistance in sub-Saharan Africa, Asia and the Near East, Latin America and the Caribbean, and Europe and Eurasia. With headquarters in Washington, D.C., USAID's strength is its field offices in many regions of the world. The agency operates in approximately one hundred developing countries, working with private voluntary organizations, indigenous groups, universities, American businesses, international organizations, other governments, trade and professional associations, faith-based organizations, and other U.S. government agencies.

Today, USAID furthers U.S. foreign policy objectives by supporting economic growth, agriculture, and trade; global health; and democracy, conflict prevention, and humanitarian assistance. USAID's core objective to improve global health includes child, maternal, and reproductive health, and the reduction of diseases such as HIV/AIDS, malaria, and tuberculosis. Nutrition interventions are key components to all of these global health objectives.

USAID's Global Nutrition Programs

More than half of the 9.7 million child deaths worldwide are linked to undernutrition. Nearly one-third of children in the developing world are chronically malnourished, and 2 billion people suffer from micronutrient deficiencies. Vitamin A deficiency affects more than 254 million children, impairing their immune systems and causing blindness, morbidity, and early mortality. Iron deficiency is the primary cause of anemia, which is responsible for 22% of maternal deaths and 24% of perinatal deaths. Today, rising prices for staple foods are causing a global food and nutrition crisis that have plunged another 130 million people into hunger and food insecurity and severely threatening progress toward improving child and maternal survival in developing countries.

Undernourished children are more likely to die than well-nourished children. Undernutrition weakens the immune response, exacerbating the effects of childhood illness such as diarrhea, measles, and pneumonia. The physical and cognitive effects of undernutrition in the first two years of life are irreversible, leading to impaired educational performance in childhood and reduced economic productivity in adulthood. The nutritional status of a pregnant woman is a deciding factor in maternal and neonatal survival. Malnutrition also exacerbates the burden of infectious diseases by increasing the susceptibility to contracting an infectious disease and by decreasing chances of survival thereafter.

USAID's nutrition strategy focuses on the following four evidence-based intervention areas:

1. Infant and young child feeding: USAID works with countries to deliver a package of key infant and child feeding interventions, including promotion of immediate initiation of breastfeeding, exclusive breastfeeding through six months of age, appropriate and high-quality complementary feeding from

six to twenty-four months, continued feeding during illness, and safe feeding practices for infants affected by HIV.

2. Micronutrient supplementation: USAID strengthens national twice-yearly vitamin A supplementation programs for children under age five through sustainable delivery mechanisms. USAID combats anemia through comprehensive anemia reduction packages, including improved iron intake, deworming, and malaria control in high-prevalence settings.

3. Food fortification: USAID helps countries introduce and expand the reach of mass fortification of staple foods with multiple micronutrients. USAID's strategic approach to mass food fortification involves both the public and private sectors.

4. Epidemics and emergencies: USAID's food security strategy addresses food access, utilization, quality, and availability to combat undernutrition. USAID supports the effective integration of community management of acute malnutrition (CMAM) into national health systems. USAID strengthens nutritional care and support for people living with HIV/AIDS and improves food assistance and food security programming in the context of HIV.

Existing Knowledge Management Tools at USAID

There are several knowledge management systems in place at USAID. The USAID Development Experience Clearinghouse (DEC) is the largest online resource for USAID-funded technical and program documentation. All USAID-funded projects are required to submit semiannual and annual reports to this system, and it currently contains more than 58,000 documents that are all available to the public.

USAID's Knowledge Services Center provides a comprehensive hub for library services, including research assistance, access to electronic databases, language training materials, and several noteworthy sources of statistics. One provides high-level data on funding for individual countries by sector. Another displays a wealth of information on demographics, population, and health (including nutrition) for every country in which USAID has a presence.

It also should be noted that with the creation of the director of foreign assistance in 2006, all U.S. government agencies have streamlined the process of planning for, tracking, and demonstrating performance of our global- and country-level investments by fiscal year. While this process is still evolving, it has already resulted in a system that USAID uses to track specific high-level results within global health and other major sectors and to create targets for upcoming years. This system is used primarily at high levels in the State Department and USAID to demonstrate success, to plan programs, and track budget levels.

There are many other tools, all of which have discrete purposes, which serve as part of USAID's wider knowledge management efforts. The key piece missing in all of them is the ability to display, record, track, and ultimately analyze all of the information flexibly so that it suits our purpose each and every time. Many times what is most useful for our daily work is a combination of all of these systems based on the type of information we need to analyze—yet the existing systems do not talk to each other. In addition, because they are entrenched and most are meant for an agency-wide audience, these systems are not easily adapted from a structural standpoint.

Nutrition Division Knowledge Management Systems

In USAID/Washington, there is a seven-person technical team working in the Global Health Bureau as part of the Nutrition Division. This team manages several centrally funded projects on the technical interventions discussed above. These projects are global in scope—with priority countries in Asia, Africa, and Latin America.

USAID has made investments in improving global nutrition over the past three decades. The success of these nutrition programs at the macro level is reductions in child mortality, achieved by innovative programs that can be adapted and replicated in other countries. With increasingly robust monitoring and evaluation systems in place, tracking short-, medium-, and long-term results has become more realistic.

Yet at the global level, facilitating the storage and use of all of these indicators of programmatic effectiveness—baseline data, results, factors of program implementation, country context, trend data—is increasingly complicated. In order to determine the success of certain programs and to learn from the challenges of others, it is imperative that USAID comprehensively track all of this information. And while USAID has a country presence in many countries and combats nutrition in a subset of these, we must also be aware of other, "nonpriority" country-level indicators in order to determine when our priorities may need to be adjusted.

Malnutrition exacerbates virtually all diseases that cause early death in developing countries—including postpartum hemorrhage, diarrhea, measles, malaria, pneumonia, HIV/AIDS, and tuberculosis. Because of this, it also is important to look at the burden of these diseases in selected countries.

There are two phases of the Nutrition Division's knowledge management effort. The second is still in process, but represents an attempt to learn from the challenges with the first system.

Initially, the knowledge management system began as an attempt to track USAID's nutrition work by technical intervention area and by centrally funded project. For example, the system could be organized by anemia reduction programs, the projects that work in the area, the countries that project is active in, and the baseline indicators for any anemia in women and children in that country. Called the Portfolio Review Management System (PRMS), it was designed in Access with the Windows.net framework, and could track a variety of interventions, countries, and indicators (see Figure 7.1).

The user interface made the system more self-explanatory and offered the opportunity to train those who may not be Access-savvy (see Figure 7.2).

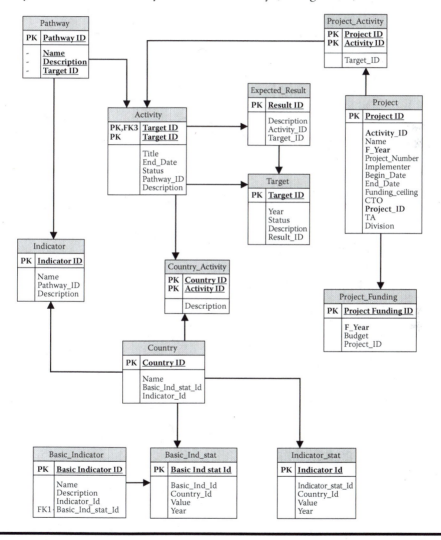

Figure 7.1 PRMS schema.

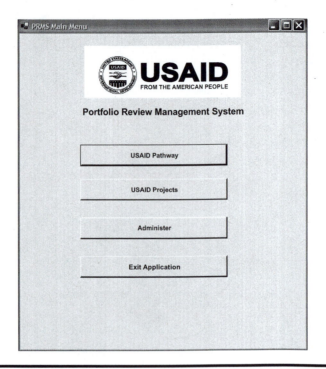

Figure 7.2 PRMS user interface.

However, there were substantial limitations to the system.

- Given the necessary security procedures for operating on USAID informa-tion technology systems, anything outside of the Microsoft Office Suite can cause problems. The Windows.net framework turned out to be a major chal-lenge to set up on USAID's server. Since the first iteration of the system was built in Access with Windows.net as the visual interface, the system had no utility without Windows.net. Even when we did obtain Windows.net, it only was available on one computer in the division.
- While some technical intervention areas remain the same from year to year, like vitamin A supplementation programs for children under five, many change. The system was not flexible enough to manipulate the technical intervention areas yet still maintain the integrity of the data behind it.
- It also became apparent that the system would replicate some of the moni-toring and evaluation work already under way by USAID's global projects. In our fast-paced work environment, any replication is an unnecessary time commitment—one that none on the technical team can make time for.
- In any knowledge management system, one must maintain the push-pull dynamic. While in the start-up phase, training will need to occur in the use and mainte-nance of a knowledge management system. Those who may not be considered

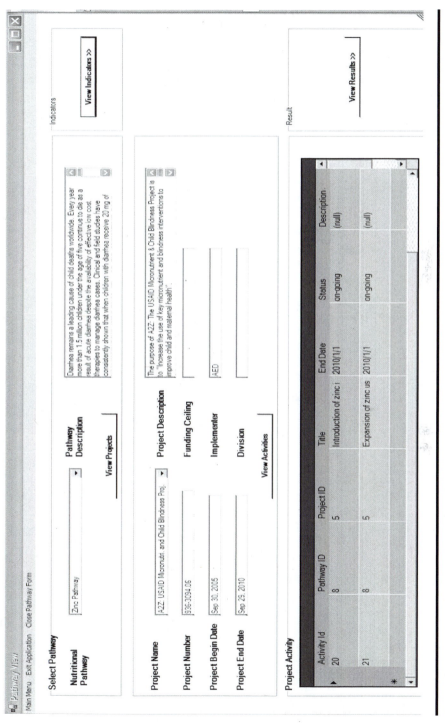

Figure 7.2 (continued)   PRMS user interface.

early adopters will need to be pushed into using a new and different system. But a successful system will inherently generate a "pull"—that is, once users understand the purpose of the system and the use of it, they should be convinced of its utility and see the potential for improving their own effectiveness. After training key members of the nutrition team (even those who tend to be early adopters), it was evident that the "pull" would not exist. There was an imbalance between maintaining the system and the potential for usefulness in our daily jobs.

■ From year to year, USAID is required to report on similar indicators to track progress in each of our programs. These indicators are often higher level, and the technical staff needs access to detailed data reports. On a weekly basis, we receive requests for data and information that is rarely the same, or in the same context, as a previous request. The purpose of the original system was to provide this detailed data in a way that could be manipulated to generate a report based on the specific request for indicators. But given the limitations of the system in terms of flexibility and manipulation, it could not provide this needed function.

■ This system was USAID-program focused, which presented two distinct challenges. One, part of the objective was to identify countries or technical areas that had gaps where USAID should focus. But the system that was constructed focused on existing interventions in existing focus countries, which made the gaps less apparent. Second, USAID-funded projects already track much of this information. While a feat to pull all of this together, it became apparent that as the system grew, it created more repetition.

In sum, perhaps the biggest fault of PRMS was that its goals, per USAID direction, were too lofty. Our biggest lesson learned was that a knowledge management system in the USAID environment cannot be the answer to every problem. In tracking by pathway (intervention area) and by USAID-supported project, we lost some of the flexibility we needed around indicators and country specifics.

But the lessons learned from the original system were a valuable starting point for building a new system, one that would suit the team's needs, require little maintenance, and return information efficiently and flexibly. This new system is being developed by technical team members, and while still in the design stages, it has already demonstrated its utility.

Based on the knowledge from PRMS that it would be difficult to have the system answer every question from both a technical and statistical standpoint, we decided to focus on the statistical side. Thus, the design of the system centers on countries, and is based on global child health, maternal health, and nutrition indicators. The biggest change from the original system was the organization around technical intervention areas. While useful to include, the changing nature of these and the degree to which regular technical input was required to ensure the accuracy of the system made it nearly impossible to make these the center of any knowledge system.

USAID's world revolves around tracking key nutrition indicators. At a basic level, USAID is held accountable for programmatic progress, and future budget levels are determined based on the achievement or lack of that success. But more importantly, diligent results tracking helps the division decide to continue supporting an approach with an eye to scale up or to reconsider an intervention in a certain country context. All USAID-supported nutrition programs have substantial monitoring and evaluation components, many of which are based on intensive work in focus districts of targeted countries.

There are multiple layers to the division's knowledge management system. The root of the system lies in tracking the following core global indicators from multiple sources:

- Under five mortality rate: Deaths between birth and the fifth birthday, expressed as deaths per 1,000 births.
- Infant mortality rate: Deaths between birth and the first birthday, expressed as deaths per 1,000 births.
- Maternal mortality rate: Maternal deaths that occur during pregnancy, childbirth, or within two months after the birth or termination of pregnancy.
- Stunting: Percentage of children under five years of age below -2 SD height for age.
- Wasting: Percentage of children under five years of age below -2 SD weight for height.
- Underweight: Percentage of children under five years of age below -2 SD weight for age.
- Vitamin A supplementation: Percentage of children six to fifty-nine months given a vitamin A supplement twice yearly.
- Anemia: Any anemia, measured by hemoglobin in children <11 g/dl and in women of reproductive age <12 g/dl.
- Household coverage of adequately iodized salt: Proportion of households consuming adequately iodized salt (fifteen parts per million or more).
- Infant and Young Child Feeding Practices: Percentage of children age six to twenty-three months who were fed according to three IYCF practices—continued breastfeeding, feeding at least the minimum number of times per day (according to age), and feeding from the minimum number of food groups per day.
- Exclusive breastfeeding: Percentage of children exclusively breastfed in the first six months of life.

The key element of the indicators database is its ability to display the same indicator from multiple data sources. USAID has conducted the demographic and health surveys in more than seventy-five countries. But these surveys only occur in selected countries and every five years. In order to make appropriate technical decisions about a nutrition technical intervention package in a selected country, other data sources are required. Major global organizations, such as the United Nations Children's Fund (UNICEF) and the World Health Organization (WHO), are other sources of data contained in our system.

In addition to the above indicators, the system tracks specific nutrition and health activities in each country, based on USAID's priorities. The historical support USAID has provided to certain countries has been critical in reducing child and maternal mortality rates. For the purposes of reporting macro-level results over the course of decades, and to track the big picture program successes and challenges, the system attempts to retrospectively present intervention areas from Global Health Bureau-supported projects from the past.

For example, USAID has long supported interventions that improve micronutrient malnutrition. The current project, called the A2Z Micronutrient and Child Blindness Project, builds on and strengthens approaches supported in the past. So the system tracks country-based and global efforts for projects supported as early as 1993 (for micronutrients, OMNI 1993–1999, MOST 1999–2005, A2Z 2005–2010) in an effort to more cohesively communicate our longstanding micronutrient interventions.

While those on the USAID nutrition team who have been with the agency for more than twenty years understand the evolution of the micronutrient portfolio, the system documents it (or at least attempts to). One can easily see that nearly all of the countries supported under OMNI focused on vitamin A supplementation, with OMNI beginning to focus on technical leadership around food fortification. MOST supported vitamin A supplementation while incorporating new interventions like zinc for treatment of diarrhea and strategic directions in maternal anemia. And today's project, A2Z, has a diverse portfolio that builds on all of this past work (both the successes and challenges): sustaining high vitamin A supplementation coverage in key countries, introducing and expanding maternal anemia packages, strengthening food fortification mechanisms at both a country and regional level, and providing technical leadership around the introduction of child anemia packages. It is rather difficult for knowledge management systems to achieve the goal of describing an organization's evolution, but by capturing these historical investments, the nutrition system makes an effort to tell this story.

Of course, the system represents nutrition as a whole, not simply micronutrients. For instance, it contains data spanning the last decade on infant and young child nutrition—including complementary feeding and breastfeeding—that are linked with USAID-funded projects LINKAGES (1996–2006) and the Infant and Young Child Nutrition Project (2006–11).

While the system does focus on data, as opposed to other knowledge management systems with a document focus, it still contains information and resources to complement the data. Recently, the nutrition system was put to the test. The Nutrition Division is involved in the president's response to the global food challenge. For the past two years, food prices have increased dramatically, presenting a major food and nutrition insecurity problem in most—if not all—of the countries USAID works in.

In a short period of time, the nutrition team needed to prioritize countries to focus on from a food security and nutrition perspective. Many factors needed to be considered to provide thoughtful analysis. We needed to balance rates of child undernutrition (based on stunting, wasting, and underweight), rates of maternal anemia (which has a direct impact on maternal mortality), the food security classification of the country (whether food insecurity is widespread, localized, etc.), where USAID has existing programs (which would hasten the response), nutrition trends in the country (including vitamin A supplementation), and which countries are on "priority" lists in the agency (maternal and child health priority, food aid priority, etc.). It would have been a monumental task simply to gather this data and compile it for the basis of our analysis.

But since a draft system is in place, we were able to quickly make some adjustments and synthesize the information we needed into the following fact sheets (Figure 7.3).

MALAWI

NEEDS		Rank	OPPORTUNITIES	
U5MR	120	14	FY08 CSMH Funding	
U5MR Rank	32	14	FY08 Non-emergency PL 480	
MMR	1,100	6	FANTA	
Underweight	19%	25	A2Z	
Stunting	46%	8	IYCN	
Wasting	3%	26	Food Security FY08	
IYCF Practices	20.1%	7/20		
Vitamin A Supplementation	36%	18		
Children with any anemia	74%	5/16	Food Security FY09	
Women with any anemia	44.3%	11/16		
			Food Security FY10	

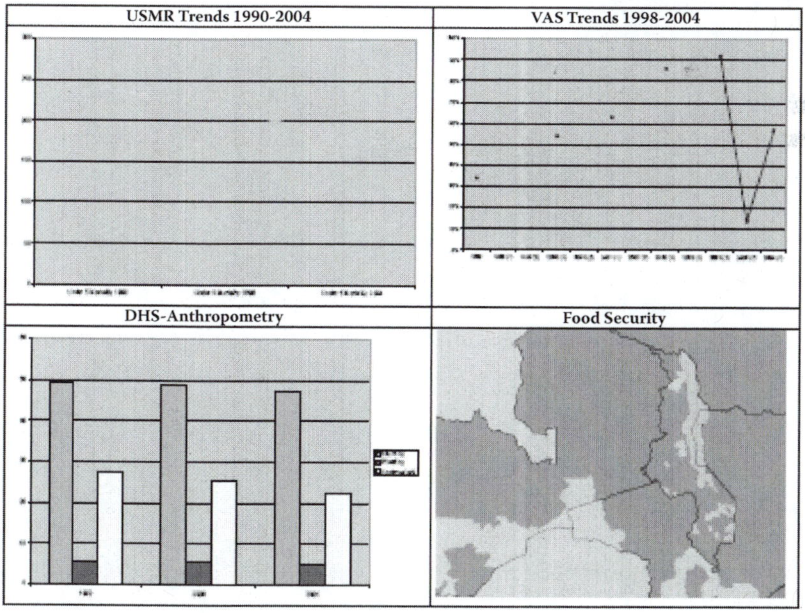

Figure 7.3   Nutrition security fact sheet for Malawi.

In addition to presenting key data points, the system was able to display information related to USAID investments and planned support (because some of this information is sensitive, it is in gray here). It also displays rankings, comparing rates of malnutrition to other maternal and child health priority countries. Given the historical nature of the system, we were able to pull trends beginning in 1990. The food security mapping is a tool developed by FEWSNET, a USAID-funded project, and is catalogued in the system. From these fact sheets, the nutrition team was able to prioritize countries based both on needs (via the indicators and rankings) and on opportunities (via existing USAID programs and planned funding priorities).

While the new system is still under development and shows promise, there are some clear limitations that will not be rectified, no matter how well designed a system is:

- Maintenance. With no administrative staff to support this effort, maintaining the relevancy and currency of the system falls on the technical team—whose members are far too busy to do so.
- Time and space. As with all knowledge management efforts, an organization must create and promote the time and space to implement such a project successfully.
- Repetition. Because there are existing systems in place, it will always be a challenge to minimize repetition and overlap.

Looking to the Future

By far our biggest immediate challenge is keeping this system up to date. In an ideal world, trends would be analyzed every six months, program information updated every quarter, and country-level statistics cleaned and verified—with new inputs—every month. To put it mildly, this is an ambitious goal and nearly impossible to implement unless the process is streamlined with minimal manual data entry.

Many knowledge management systems measure how many new documents are loaded into the system, how often it is used, how long it is used for, etc. There are no set metrics for measuring the impact of this system. Since the system was internally initiated with the purpose of making the team's daily work more efficient, the sole measure of success is that we are able to find the kind of information we need more quickly, and that that information is paired with appropriate knowledge resources, including technical interventions areas, USAID support over the decades, upcoming priorities, and past programmatic success.

The longer-term challenge is how this system becomes, or fails to become, institutionalized. USAID staff is always on a quest for knowledge; after all, it is a cornerstone of our jobs to remain current on scientific discoveries in public health and nutrition. The key will be to marry this quest for new scientific and programmatic knowledge with a more thoughtful understanding of the current and historical state of nutrition and USAID's role at a global and country scale.

As Davenport et al. state in their review of successful knowledge management efforts, "effective knowledge management is neither panacea nor bromide." USAID's nutrition team has learned this from the past year and several iterations of a system. Our challenge now is to ensure its use and longevity through proven utility in our daily work environment. That will not be the sole measure of success, but perhaps the most valuable.

Chapter 8

Formulating KM Strategies at the Local Level

A New Approach to Knowledge Sharing in Large Public Health Organizations

Richard Van West-Charles and Arthur J. Murray

Contents

Background

This chapter documents the activities, accomplishments, and lessons learned of a knowledge management (KM) transformation initiative undertaken by the Information and Knowledge Management (IKM) Area of the Pan American Health Organization (PAHO), one of six regional components comprising the World Health Organization (WHO).

Since its inception more than one hundred years ago in response to the threat of mosquito-borne and drinking water-related illnesses during the construction of the Panama Canal, PAHO has been a knowledge-intensive organization. The term "technical cooperation," which appears frequently in its mission and policy documents, underlies its role in providing specialized expertise in response to public health concerns across the region.

For most of its history, these concerns were relatively narrow in scope. Outbreaks of foot-and-mouth disease were handled by specialists in that particular field of veterinary public health. Denge fever had its own team of specialists, and so forth. This gave rise to an organizational structure consisting of numerous silos, each focused on a particular disease or discipline.

For most of the twentieth century, this structure performed adequately. However, the twenty-first century ushered in a new era of speed and complexity. The U.N. Millennium Development Goals (MDGs) were created to address a variety of global issues, including public health. For example, combating the spread of HIV/AIDS involves specialties ranging from public relations and education to population studies, to modeling and simulation, to the production and administration of serums and associated treatment protocols.

Even more illustrative of the paradigm shift in public health was the threat of avian flu. The isolated incidents of potential outbreaks which occurred in the mid-2000s time frame revealed that many different components of the organization, which used to operate in isolation, had to openly collaborate and share knowledge in order to deal with this new type of threat.

The H5N1 virus is carried by migratory species, and can quickly and unexpectedly mutate. Vaccines cannot be developed until the jump is made to humans. But the disease spreads so quickly it outpaces the ability to mass produce vaccines and antivirals in a timely fashion. Rapid response is the key to detection and containment, and requires the ability to properly collect, package, and ship specimens across international borders for testing, all within forty-eight hours or less. Proper means for dealing with the news media in a timely manner, in order to keep the population educated and informed without creating a panic, are essential. All of these actions require *knowledge*, which necessitates a new paradigm of large-scale collaboration and knowledge sharing.

This chapter addresses how the transformation to this new paradigm was accomplished, including the breaking down of longstanding silos, and the emergence of online communities of practice and virtual workspaces for dealing with these rapidly changing and complex threats.

The Desired End State

The overarching goal of the transformation program was to help PAHO become an organization characterized by the following four states:

1. An authoritative source on health information and knowledge
2. An effective collaboration-based organization
3. A learning organization
4. A partnership and network-building organization

In other words, the goal was to transition PAHO from a traditional, knowledge-hoarding organization into a twenty-first-century knowledge-sharing enterprise. The knowledge-hoarding organization is characterized by silos that are heavily guarded and protected. Any knowledge that does flow often occurs in informal settings, such as the cafeteria, or the smoking area outside the building, or around the printer or water cooler. Silos are further reinforced by well-meaning but rigid work processes and management systems, as well as by an underlying labyrinth of disparate information technology (IT) systems and applications.

In the goal state, the formal organization, although still present, moves into the background, and the social network becomes prominent. Rather than hiding in the shadows, the network "sees" itself, and therefore "knows" itself. Enabled by tools such as social network analysis, the channels through which critical knowledge is exchanged become transparent.

In addition to a more visible social network, the learning cycle of developing, sharing, and applying knowledge becomes formalized and embedded within every work process. Finally, silos cannot be removed if the IT architecture itself remains fragmented. Instead, IT needs to evolve into a services-oriented architecture (SOA) in which data, business logic, and applications are compatible, enabling the rapid exchange of knowledge across the enterprise.

Once these key change elements come together, the old "in-the-shadows" form of knowledge sharing begins to dissipate, and the development, sharing, and application of knowledge occur more by design, rather than by chance. This illustrates the end state toward which the local KM strategies were targeted. The approach to developing and implementing those strategies, and the results observed, will be presented next.

Transformation Approach

The basic approach of the transformation initiative was intentionally kept simple: to provide education and guidance through a series of workshops and online content in:

1. Organizing and activating communities of practice (CoPs) in selected technical cooperation areas
2. Providing a methodology for each CoP to formulate and implement its own KM strategy

This represents an important shift in typical KM practices. In many large organizations, executive management, such as the chief knowledge officer (CKO), dictates a KM strategy, which the entire enterprise is obliged to follow. This approach is not appropriate for large, multidisciplinary, geographically dispersed organizations such as PAHO.

Since PAHO's reach extends far beyond its Washington, D.C., headquarters into remote villages of economically disadvantaged countries, the resources available for developing, sharing, and applying knowledge vary greatly from country to country. More importantly, some of the most critical knowledge is developed, and has its most direct application, in the field. For this reason, *the transformation approach we employed was focused on educating the workforce and empowering the practitioners with the tools they needed to leverage critical knowledge in the most effective way.*

This meant each community had to develop and execute its own KM strategy. Since this ultimately required a change in work processes and behaviors, an essential part of the approach was ensuring that members of the workforce understood why they needed to change, and how a local KM strategy, and the application of various KM tools and practices, would help make their lives easier.

Determining Which Knowledge Is Critical to Mission Success

Our experience demonstrated that, in order to be successful, any KM initiative must be in direct alignment with the organization's mission. For this reason, throughout the transformation program, the overall goal was to help PAHO achieve its stated mission: *To lead strategic collaborative efforts among Member States and other partners to promote equity in health, to combat disease, and to improve the quality of, and lengthen, the lives of the peoples of the Americas.*

Most knowledge capture efforts are wasted, as organizations attempt to capture any and all knowledge available. Some even go to great lengths to interview key personnel who are planning to transfer or retire. The key question is, *What knowledge do we really need?* Capturing all of an organization's knowledge is impractical,

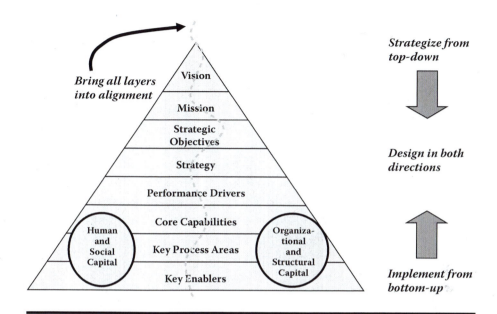

Figure 8.1 A strategic flow-down approach which aligns people, processes, and technology.

if not impossible. On the opposite end of the spectrum, some organizations try to capture knowledge opportunistically, as problems or issues arise. The risk of that approach is that the most valuable knowledge may not be discovered until a crisis occurs, which may be too late.

Our approach was to implement a "drill-down" process, in which we identified the critical knowledge needed for PAHO to achieve its desired level of mission success (see Figure 8.1). The drill-down flowed from PAHO's vision and mission, to its strategic objectives, to the strategy for achieving those objectives. Once the strategy was understood, we identified the key performance drivers needed to successfully accomplish the strategy. Next, we identified the core capabilities needed to achieve the desired level of performance and the key process areas which make up those core capabilities. Finally, we identified the tangible and intangible assets needed to execute the key processes in the most efficient and effective way.

Being a knowledge enterprise, the majority of PAHO's assets are intangible, consisting of:

■ Human capital: Achieving sustained high performance through continuous learning and innovation, and the development of skills and competencies for doing so, while remaining focused on key performance drivers.
■ Social capital: Focusing not on *what* you know or *who* you know, but rather on what you know *about* whom you know.

- Organizational capital: Improving efficiency and effectiveness through streamlined, self-managed processes.
- Structural capital: Ensuring smooth communication and integration across all organizational elements and systems.

The output product of this drill-down exercise was a KM strategy for each organizational unit, based on an optimal combination of people, processes and technologies, all operating in a way that maximized the flow of knowledge throughout the enterprise. This process revealed and allowed us to address the major obstacles and barriers preventing attainment of the goals and objectives, including cultural, political, financial, interorganizational, intraorganizational, and many other issues.

Many KM projects begin by looking at the large volumes of information in an organization, then attempting to identify how best to use them. But true knowledge management deals with the correct *application* of information. For an organization such as PAHO, this means choosing the right course of action. By focusing on enhancing and streamlining critical decision processes, scarce resources (people, time, and dollars) could be applied more efficiently and effectively.

Approach for Developing the Local KM Strategies

Since its inception, the discipline of knowledge management has suffered from confusion and resistance, brought about by trainers who make the subject too complex and too difficult to understand in a practical way. Practitioners, although they may be somewhat interested in KM, have very little time and patience for academically oriented transformation programs. For this reason, we used a four-step KM approach that was very basic and easy to understand:

Step 1. Identify the desired results

- *Who* is involved?
- *What* is the result?
- *When* does it happen?
- *Where?*
- *Why?*
- *How* is the result to be achieved?

Step 2. Assess the current process, and identify the gaps

- What is working well, and why?
- What isn't working (gaps)?

Step 3. Determine if the principles of KM can close the gaps

- Developing knowledge: Has the right knowledge been identified and captured so it can be reused?
- Sharing knowledge: Is the right knowledge being made available to those who need it, when they need it?
- Applying knowledge: Is the right knowledge being used consistently, in the right way?

Step 4. Develop and implement a KM Strategy

- Engaging the right people
- Streamlining and enhancing work processes
- Enabling technologies

This resulting strategy can be represented in a simple diagram, shown in Figure 8.2.

Pilot Implementation

Next, we initiated the search for a pilot group. The ideal group needed to be a diverse, multidisciplinary community that illustrated and exemplified the need for breaking down silos and sharing knowledge.

At that point in time, the possibility of an outbreak of pandemic influenza was a major concern. This turned out to be an excellent motivator for change. It demanded close collaboration and rapid communication among many diverse disciplines, which had been previously functioning in isolation. These included veterinary public health; communicable diseases; communications and media; immunology; epidemiology; the production, distribution, and administering of vaccines and antiviral drugs; and crisis response planning, including the use of modeling and simulation.

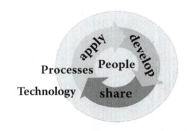

Figure 8.2   Key components of a localized KM strategy.

An emergency action response (EAR) task force was formed, and its members were trained in the KM strategy development methodology. After a short period of time, it became obvious that the group was too large. Discussions regarding specific issues, although important, left many participants on the periphery of the conversation. The group was quickly divided into five subgroups, which became more manageable. Discussions continued to focus on specific areas, while not losing sight of the broader picture. The five subgroups were the following:

1. Communications
2. Health care services
3. Preparedness
4. Prevention
5. Surveillance

Building a Virtual Environment for Developing, Sharing, and Applying Knowledge

At the outset of the transformation initiative, PAHO's knowledge portal was under development, using the Microsoft SharePoint Portal Services® platform. Like many organizations, the portal was mainly used as an electronic document library. XML metadata tags, along with search tools, were used to categorize and label documents, in the hope of providing insight into what knowledge was contained in the collection. But users still had to spend a great deal of time poring through text, seeking relevant information, and extracting the knowledge. Worse yet, much of the knowledge being sought was implicit and not even in the system.

As we mentioned earlier, the most valuable organizational knowledge was found in casual conversations, "war stories," and the like. Figure 8.3 illustrates this notion, contrasting the scarcity of knowledge in documents and reports with the richness of knowledge in stories and conversations.

To meet the public health challenges of a rapidly changing world, a new, innovative approach to developing, sharing, and applying knowledge was needed: an approach that is truly knowledge-centric, not document-centric. Such an approach recognizes that knowledge is exchanged primarily in stories, conversations, and actions, rather than in documents. We addressed this problem by encouraging and reinforcing a change in mindset, from documents to knowledge "nuggets." The new mindset is illustrated in Figure 8.4.

Knowledge nuggets can take many forms, from "fast facts" and vignettes, to blog postings, even trip report summaries. We incorporated this new mindset in our redesign of the traditional portal into a more knowledge-centric portal, as

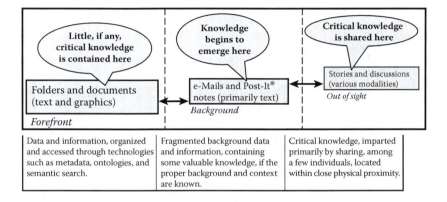

Figure 8.3 Current approaches focus on documents, with knowledge in the background.

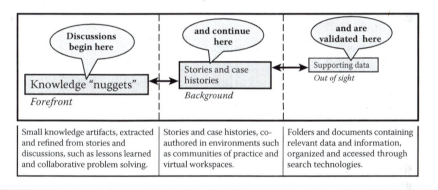

Figure 8.4 New approaches move knowledge to the foreground, supported by documents.

illustrated in Figure 8.5. Note that the new portal was bilingual, which greatly expanded the reach and level of participation.

A facility for initiating and conducting online collaborative discussions was implemented on the left-hand side of Figure 8.5, labeled "Discussions." The discussions were advanced by adding supporting data and analysis, and even anecdotal evidence, such as stories and vignettes. This was performed in the area labeled "Stories and Lessons Learned." Finally, when the community accepted the claims along with the supporting evidence, the knowledge was formally published in the area on the right labeled "Best Practices." Note the "e-Library" tab, which kept the supporting data and documents within reach, while not taking up valuable real estate on the CoP home page. Overall, this provided a simple, yet effective, way of

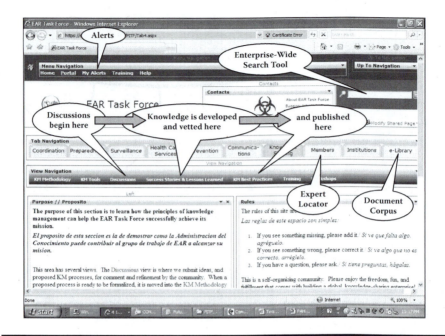

Figure 8.5 A SharePoint portal configuration which supports the knowledge life cycle.

using a common infrastructure tool, Microsoft SharePoint®, and adapting it to support the paradigm shift from focusing on documents to focusing on knowledge.

Knowledge Validation

An important issue was periodically raised: *What degree of knowledge validation is appropriate?* On one hand, if a structured, albeit well-meaning, knowledge vetting process is imposed, the frequency of knowledge sharing can decrease dramatically. On the other hand, in an organization such as PAHO, in which serious public health risks may be at stake, a vetting process is warranted. The question was, how best to balance open participation versus validation?

The answer was dependent upon the type of knowledge being developed, shared, and applied. Consider, for example, a situation in which a serious pandemic is under way, and resources such as vaccines, or even syringes, are in short supply. Although the temptation may be great to find innovative ways to stretch limited resources, care must be taken to safeguard against administering incorrect dosages, or taking shortcuts in areas such as using sterilized equipment. While such measures may seem to make sense in the short run, especially in terms of alleviating the immediate crisis, they may cause more serious long-term effects.

On the other hand, not all situations demand careful vetting. In fact, in many situations, a long vetting process could exact a heavy toll. For example, an on-the-spot decision was made in Buenos Aries, Argentina, to open the HIV/AIDS counseling centers during late-night hours. By taking decisive action, and quickly sharing the results, a positive impact was made in the number of at-risk individuals seeking counseling. If this knowledge nugget were withheld in order to go through a long validation process, it would have caused unreasonable and unnecessary delays in the fight against HIV/AIDS.

That is not to say that the knowledge can be applied everywhere. For example, in some countries, late-night operations may be in violation of curfews or other laws, and could have serious consequences for the counselors and their organization. Still, such exceptions could be more quickly identified in an "open" knowledge-sharing system, as opposed to one that has a rigid, tightly controlled validation cycle.

Expanse of Reach

Approximately four hundred people participated in the strategy development program at various stages. This included ninety-eight registered participants in the five EAR task force groups. The initiative exhibited the multiplier effects of a "train-the trainer" approach, resulting in a broad reach across PAHO. Each group participating in a workshop had one or more individuals willing to carry the banner, and help others in their community by showing them how to use the tools, and acting as a catalyst to get others to participate. This produced even greater leverage throughout the organization.

The effort also received tremendous leverage through the mentoring of Information and Knowledge Management (IKM) interns, who in turn provided mentoring and technical assistance to CoP members in the development of their KM strategies and in the use of the various tools. Communications across the organization helped to maintain high visibility into the effort. Directors, areas managers, and unit chiefs were periodically informed of progress, and outstanding and notable efforts of individuals were recognized.

Overall Evaluation of the KM Approach

Throughout the transformation program, periodic surveys and questionnaires were administered. More than 100 responses were received and catalogued. In summary, the KM strategies which were applied to the various CoPs, and the approach to developing those strategies, exhibited the following characteristics:

1. Proven applicability across domains. The basic four-step strategy development approach was used effectively in a variety of domains, covering a wide cross-section of the PAHO organization, both functionally and geographically. Legacy groups, formerly operating in silos, were brought together, but usually after a common goal was articulated and well understood. Although language in general proved not to be a barrier, terminology specific to various groups did occasionally pose a problem. This required a concerted effort by each group to better understand the other groups' terminology. Once this happened, the knowledge began to flow more freely across the various domains.

2. Varying degrees of acceptance. In every group, there consistently emerged one or two individuals who were extremely excited about the possibility of change and how knowledge management could help their organization. These individuals often served as catalysts who helped to build and sustain the momentum necessary for change. By the same token, there were usually one or two individuals on the other side of the spectrum who were very skeptical. The remainder of each group was mostly in between, "sitting on the fence." These individuals, although not completely sold on the idea, were at least open to the possibility of change. Once the one or two catalysts in the group began to put the principles into practice, the middle of the group began to see the benefits, and slowly started adopting the principles and practices themselves.

3. Increased mission effectiveness through the use of KM tools. A main concern which repeatedly appeared was *workload*. Most people see themselves as overworked, overburdened, and underpaid. Consequently, they look at any new initiative, including KM, as a burden. The problem is compounded because most new tools and practices require training, which also is viewed as a waste of time. The challenge, therefore, was to clearly demonstrate that doing things the old way was unacceptable, and a greater drain on one's time than doing things the new way.

   A simple example of this was the introduction of a knowledge mapping tool. While it took an investment of time to build the map, most people understood the benefit of being able to visually capture how everything was interconnected, significantly reducing the amount of time that would have been lost by not involving the right people in planning and decision processes.

4. Demonstrated ability to apply the principles of KM in everyday practice. The basic notion of developing, sharing, and applying knowledge was a powerful tool in helping people understand how to apply the principles of KM. Another strong concept was the notion of identifying the gaps. Once people understood the benefit of viewing problems from the standpoint of knowledge gaps, and applying the develop-share-apply cycle as a means of closing the gaps, the incorporation of KM into everyday work processes gradually became habitual. This is the only way a true learning organization can ultimately be created.

Conclusions

Focusing on real results and tangible improvements in performance was instrumental in reinforcing behavioral change. The use of metrics indicated whether organizational learning was occurring, and whether each new initiative was an improvement over the previous one. Some notable performance indicators that were used included the following:

- The ability to respond more quickly to changes or requests
- The ability to make business decisions faster, better, and more consistently
- Increased productivity
- Improved morale and increased passion about one's work and contribution to the overall mission
- Cost reductions realized from making fewer errors and eliminating redundant activities

In summary, empowering smaller organizational units to develop and implement their own KM strategy greatly enhanced the ability of a large, multinational institution to generate, share, and apply knowledge across the enterprise. From directors and managers at the headquarters level to practitioners in the field, the formation of virtual communities around specific problem areas or disciplines provided an effective and efficient means of responding to the public health challenges of a complex, rapidly changing world.

Acknowledgments

The work cited in this chapter was funded under PAHO Service Contract SC-05-02494. The authors also wish to acknowledge Drs. Francesco Calabrese and Alfredo Revilak of the Enterprise Excellence Management Group Inc., who actively contributed to the success of the transformation initiative.

Chapter 9

Knowledge Management

*A Mechanism for Promoting
Evidence-Informed Public
Health Decision Making*

Maureen Dobbins, Paula Robeson,
Kara DeCorby, Heather Husson, Daiva Trillis,
Edwin Lee, and Lori Greco

Contents

Introduction

Evidence-Informed Public Health

It is generally believed that research evidence, if effectively transferred, could inform policy and practice decisions and subsequently improve health outcomes (1). Evidence-informed decision making (EIDM) involves the incorporation of the best available evidence from a systematically collected, appraised, and analyzed body of knowledge (2–4). Each step of the process requires unique skills and knowledge, which have been shown to be limited among public health professionals (5, 6). Furthermore, barriers such as time greatly reduce the extent to which decision makers engage in EIDM. The literature demonstrates that knowledge translation and exchange (KTE) strategies, which overcome time and limited capacity to identify, appraise, and synthesize evidence, hold promise for promoting EIDM (7–9). The ultimate goal of KTE activities is to facilitate the incorporation of research knowledge into the decision-making process and ultimately policies, practice, and eventually health outcomes. The term implies that effective strategies are all that are needed to achieve this end. It all appears so rational, logical, and, well, simple. So, why has it proved so challenging to achieve EIDM among public health organizations and decision makers? Furthermore, would we know if we had achieved it?

Knowledge Management in Public Health

Knowledge management (KM) is emerging as a key factor in the realization of evidence-informed public health practice (10–12). KM comprises a range of practices used by organizations to identify, create, represent, distribute, and enable adoption of what it knows, and how it knows it (13, 14). KM may be distinguished from organizational learning by a greater focus on the management of knowledge as an asset and the development and cultivation of the channels through which knowledge and information flow (15, 16). KM always has existed in one form or another. However, it has been most prominent in the private sector, and specifically the technology sector, and is relatively new as a field of research. While its relevance and importance for public health practice have been acknowledged, currently little is understood or developed about effective KM processes (14). KM activities often are guided by knowledge taxonomies to organize what is known, how it is known, and its potential use(s) (14, 17, 18). Examples include on-the-job peer discussions, formal apprenticeship, discussion forums, corporate libraries, professional training, and mentoring programs (12, 18). With computers becoming more widespread in the second half of the twentieth century, specific adaptations of technology, such as knowledge repositories, have been introduced to further enhance the process (17). However, there is a need to ensure that KM systems are held to the same standard that is applied to empirical research. That means that KM systems should be based on appropriate theoretical paradigms, be transparent, utilize rigorous methods, and be evidence based themselves. This chapter discusses two key concepts of KM as it relates to public health practice. The first involves the description of a public health knowledge repository, including what it is, how it was developed, and how it is being used. The second involves a description of one way in which this KM system, quickly and with minimal resources, addressed an important information need identified by medical officers of health in one province in Canada. The overall aim of this initiative was to facilitate the translation of the best available research evidence on chronic disease prevention into public health policy and program planning.

Background

While there are some systematic reviews regarding strategies to change health care practitioner behavior (19–21), there are currently no definitive answers of how best to move toward "evidence-informed" public health practice. Barriers to EIDM include lack of time, limited access to research evidence, limited capacity to appraise and translate research evidence, excessive literature, unsupportive work environments, lack of decision-making authority, processes not conducive to KTE, and resistance to change (5, 7, 22–29). System-level changes that may facilitate EIDM include more effective communication of research findings to decision makers, better understanding of the context in which decision makers work, and building collaborative relationships with decision makers (1, 30–33). Furthermore, decision makers must become more receptive to including the best available research evidence in decision making, become critical consumers of research evidence, and must be willing to collaborate with researchers to ensure relevant research is conducted (34–36).

While traditional passive dissemination strategies (i.e., publications, Web sites) used alone have been shown to be ineffective in promoting EIDM (8, 37), interactive strategies involving face-to-face contact and targeting messages at specific audiences have shown promising results (7–9, 38–40). It is thought that a combination of activities that reach potential users on multiple levels may be effective in achieving EIDM (2, 41). Organizational context (27, 42–45) and the value organizations place on research evidence use are significantly associated with EIDM (28, 45, 46). Furthermore, decision-making processes and staff training in critical appraisal and research use are strongly linked to EIDM (26, 43, 47–50). These findings align closely with the concepts of knowledge management with respect to building capacity and mechanisms for facilitating the flow of information into and within the organization.

One of the emerging trends in the KTE field is the increasing use of and reliance on technology, particularly Internet-based mechanisms. Certainly the potential of the Internet to reach large numbers of decision makers is great, but can such mechanisms really facilitate the cultural shift in organizational thinking and foster sustained KTE capacity among individuals that is so necessary for system-wide change? Currently there is limited research available on the effectiveness of the Internet as a KTE strategy, even less exploring its impact on evidence-informed decision making, and almost no studies assessing impact on patient or population health outcomes. One Canadian study found that the dissemination of best practices information to public health professionals via the Internet encouraged participants to access information at other online sites compared to print-based dissemination (51). These findings are especially relevant since much of the current literature is now accessible online. Participants in this same study cited easy access to relevant information as a major benefit, saving managers from having to identify, access, and retrieve their own literature. When traveling to face-to-face meetings is not possible, the Internet also provides a valuable communication and networking opportunity for professional practice (52), while facilitating research collaboration (53).

A Knowledge Repository: Health-evidence.ca

The key premise of EIDM is the incorporation of the best available evidence from a systematically collected, appraised, and analyzed body of knowledge. Literature reviews—which encompass a rigorous and transparent process for retrieving and appraising relevant research evidence on a specific topic to determine the overall effectiveness of a given intervention, on specified outcomes, for a particular popu-lation—can be particularly powerful tools to inform and influence public health decision making and practice (54–57). Specific types of reviews include system-atic reviews, meta-analyses, meta-syntheses (58, 59), and best practice guidelines. Synthesized evidence provides a more consistent and conservative estimate of effect for interventions in comparison to individual studies, and as such is a more power-ful tool to guide practice (60–63).

Health-evidence.ca is a knowledge repository of systematic reviews evaluating public health and health promotion interventions, published since 1985. It is a KM system, developed in Canada, specifically for public health and health promotion decision makers at all levels, although it is applicable to multiple audiences, includ-ing practitioners, policymakers, research funders, students, and researchers. The goal of health-evidence.ca is to facilitate decision maker access to, retrieval of, and use of the best available research evidence, so as to promote EIDM.

Initial efforts to build this KM system began in 2000 and culminated with its launch on March 10, 2005. A number of funded studies preceding site develop-ment focused on understanding program planning decision-making processes in public health organizations (64, 65), led to the development of a knowledge uti-lization framework for public health decision makers (66), and informed the key functions and components of health-evidence.ca. In addition, a study funded by the Canadian Institutes of Health Research (CIHR), "Strategies for Disseminating Systematic Reviews in Public Health," explored Canadian public health decision makers' needs and preferences for receiving research evidence in the form of systematic reviews. Multiple methods, including telephone-administered surveys, qualitative, individual, face-to-face interviews, and focus groups were used to collect this data. Data from these studies demonstrated a strong desire among Canadian public health decision makers for a national repository of research evidence, assessed for methodological quality and which could be accessed easily online (6, 33). These findings formed the basis for the creation of health-evidence.ca.

Health-evidence.ca is one component of a broader knowledge translation and exchange strategy that supports users in accessing and interpreting research evidence, and connects users through online communities of practice. In the short term (one to three years) this KM system aimed to (a) provide an easily accessible source of published, reliable, up-to-date reviews evaluating the effectiveness of public health and health promotion interventions; (b) act as a communication tool to facilitate exchange among Canadian public health and health promotion decision makers and researchers; (c) build familiarity with the interpretation and integration of research evidence into the decision-making process; (d) provide decision makers with the tools to enhance their critical appraisal skills; (e) customize the content received by decision makers to their specified areas of interest; and (f) improve strategic networking and partnership building among researchers, decision makers, and practitioners by providing mechanisms to interact.

In the long term (five to ten years) this KM system will (a) continue to be the go-to source for published and unpublished reviews in public health and health promotion effectiveness; (b) host various online communities of practice (Canadian and international in scope) to promote knowledge translation and exchange; (c) provide a mechanism for evaluating innovative KTE strategies; and (d) provide a forum for ongoing networking among researchers and public health decision makers. The following sections will chronicle the journey of the development, launch, and maintenance of health-evidence.ca to the present time.

A good KM system provides a multitude of functions that respond directly to the needs of its intended users (67). This concept was a driving force behind the development of health-evidence.ca, with respect to particular functions and features. Embedded functions include:

- A user registration process that allows users to tailor the information they receive to particular areas of interest.
- A search system that is searchable by commonly used public health and health promotion terms.
- An assessment of the methodological quality of each review that is reported upon.
- A sorting system that allows users to sort search results by review quality (strong, moderate, or weak), topic area, intervention location, or type.
- A standardized summary template (2 pages) for each review written by public health decision makers for public health decision makers. Each summary

frames the issue and links each evidence point with implications for policy and practice.

■ A built-in feedback loop provides users with the opportunity to give suggestions on site improvement.

Creating Health-evidence.ca: Methods

Development Phase

The systematic reviews that populate health evidence.ca were identified through a comprehensive search strategy (1985–present) that included electronic searches of seven databases: MEDLINE, EMBASE, CINAHL, PsycINFO, Sociological Abstracts, BIOSIS, and SportDiscus. In addition, hand searching of more than fifty journals was undertaken, and the reference lists of all relevant reviews were examined for additional references. The review process is depicted in Figure 9.1. Abstracts from all search strategies were imported into Reference Manager and screened independently by two reviewers. Reviews judged as potentially relevant were retrieved either electronically or in hard copy and assessed for relevance by two independent reviewers using a previously developed and tested tool (available from the first author). Relevance criteria included (1) is the article a review; (2) is the intervention relevant to public health practice; (3) is the effectiveness of an intervention the focus of the review; (4) is evidence on health outcomes reported; and (5) is the search strategy described. Reviews had to meet all five criteria in order to be included in the repository. Any discrepancies in relevance ratings were resolved through consensus.

Relevant reviews were then read and keywords assigned using a tool developed by project staff through consultation with public health experts. The intent was to assign commonly used public health and health promotion terms so as to facilitate search efforts of public health decision makers. Keyword terms were categorized into the following major themes: review focus, type of review, population or age group, intervention location, and intervention strategy. The draft keyword tool was finalized by group consensus, and keywording was shared among project staff with regular meetings to review decision making and discuss appropriate assignment of terms. The application of the keywording tool was agreed upon, and generally keywording was performed by one staff member, with any issues raised discussed in a group meeting. Periodic checks of interrater agreement for keywords were conducted on a biannual basis.

Relevant reviews were then assessed for methodological quality by two independent reviewers using a previously developed and tested tool modified from an existing tool (40) and pretested for reliability (68). The ten criteria used to assess methodological quality were (1) a clearly focused question; (2) inclusion criteria explicitly stated; (3) comprehensive search strategy; (4) adequate number of years covered in the search; (5) description of level of evidence; (6) assessment of the methodological rigor of primary studies; (7) methodological quality of primary

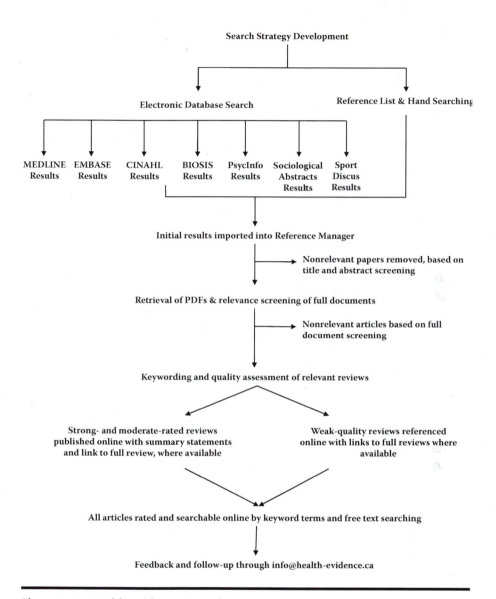

Search Strategy Development

Electronic Database Search

Reference List & Hand Searching

| MEDLINE Results | EMBASE Results | CINAHL Results | BIOSIS Results | PsycInfo Results | Sociological Abstracts Results | Sport Discus Results |

Initial results imported into Reference Manager

Nonrelevant papers removed, based on title and abstract screening

Retrieval of PDFs & relevance screening of full documents

Nonrelevant articles based on full document screening

Keywording and quality assessment of relevant reviews

Strong- and moderate-rated reviews published online with summary statements and link to full review, where available

Weak-quality reviews referenced online with links to full reviews where available

All articles rated and searchable online by keyword terms and free text searching

Feedback and follow-up through info@health-evidence.ca

Figure 9.1   Health-evidence.ca review process.

studies assessed by two reviewers and results given; (8) tests of homogeneity or assessment of similarity of results conducted and reported; (9) appropriate weighting of primary studies; and (10) author's interpretation of results supported by the data.

Each criterion, worth one point each, was given equal weight in the overall methodological assessment score. Reviews were given an overall score out of ten and were classified into three categories: strong, moderate, and weak. Reviews receiving an overall rating of seven or more were considered strong; those with a score of five or six, moderate; and those with four or less, weak. Discrepancies were resolved by discussion.

The intent was that all reviews receiving a strong or moderate quality rating (rating of five or higher out of a possible ten points) would be summarized in a concise (approximately two-page) summary statement that gives an overview of the review's content, places the review's topic and findings within a Canadian context, summarizes the methodological quality of the review in terms of consistent and well-accepted criteria, and outlines the key findings and resulting implications for policy and practice in public health, which can reasonably be drawn from the review's findings. Implications may be drawn from the review itself, providing that they are accurate and supported in the data, and may represent the views of the review author(s), or be drawn only by the summary statement author. Health-evidence.ca staff wrote summaries for reviews in which they had experience and expertise. For topics in which health-evidence.ca staff did not have the necessary expertise, public health decision makers with the relevant expertise were enlisted to write the implications sections of the summary. The goal of these short summaries is to present the results of reviews in plain language, explicitly identifying the key messages and implications for policy and practice, which could be read and interpreted in two to three minutes. For example, an effect size provided in a meta-analysis with a confidence interval or level of statistical significance (p value) was explained in terms that could be interpreted by a reader with no statistical background. The numerical data, of course, are still provided. So although the language and terminology of the reviews may vary, the language of the summary statements is consistent and easily transferable to decision makers at various levels with differing educational backgrounds and experience, thus making the summary easier to pass on and use. However, users are encouraged to consult the full review for greater detail as needed.

Each summary statement also provides a list of related reviews and resources for the reader's use. Summary statements include suggestions on how to cite the summary statement itself, as well as reference to the full review being summarized, and contact information for the first author of the reviews, wherever possible. All reviews being summarized are within the public domain, and the summary statement provides appropriate disclaimers to make the distinction between summary statement and review authorship, and that summary statement authors' views do not necessarily represent those of the review author. Health-evidence.ca also makes available links to the full reviews where they are publicly accessible online or by IP authentication if users of our site have existing journal or database (i.e., EBSCO/OVID) subscriptions. The goal is simply to catalogue and make available references to all of the published review evidence on effectiveness of public health interventions, and to provide summaries of that evidence to facilitate their use by decision makers. Summary statement writing has been largely unfunded, with the exception of a small number of projects funded to generate summaries in a particular topic area. At present more than two-thirds of reviews in health-evidence.ca still require summary statements to be written, and efforts are ongoing to secure funding to gradually reduce this number.

Health-evidence.ca provides all static content pages, such as additional resources, site information, and tools, in French as well as English; however, funding has not yet been available to translate all of the reference material in the site, nor to screen, appraise, and summarize any French-language reviews encountered in the electronic database searching. Health-evidence.ca is prioritizing the translation of summaries for well-done (strong or moderate quality) reviews housed in the registry.

Maintenance Phase

Between March 2005 and the present, the health-evidence.ca registry has been updated quarterly through ongoing electronic searches, reference list searches, and hand searches. Each quarter approximately 30,000 titles and abstracts are screened, and the set of potentially relevant reviews is reduced to approximately 250 to 300 references, which are retrieved in full text for relevance testing, keywording, and methodological quality assessment. Searches have been programmed in four of the electronic health databases (MEDLINE, EMBASE, CINAHL, and PsycINFO) to be executed automatically upon database update (every one to two weeks). Links to the automatically generated results are e-mailed to the project manager for importing and tracking of the results sets. Due to limited database features for running automated searches or limiting searches by time periods shorter than one year, the three other electronic health databases (BIOSIS, SportDiscus, and Sociological Abstracts) are searched annually. Hand searching also is done annually over the summer months, due to its human resource intensiveness and accessibility of students to assist in this activity. The reference list of each relevant review also is examined for additional potentially relevant reviews.

Each quarter, potentially relevant references are uploaded to the Web site via XML files exported from Reference Manager. An online collaboration feature of the site allows for relevance testing, keywording, and quality assessment to be completed online. The online collaboration enables a completely paperless screening and assessment process, and is not a publicly accessible component of health-evidence.ca. PDFs of reviews are uploaded and attached to each reference in the online system. Due to copyright restrictions, access to PDFs is only available to internal health-evidence.ca staff during the assessment process. Once reviews are added to the public domain, PDFs are not accessible by the public. Once a PDF is attached to a reference, the review moves to a queue for "articles requiring relevance," where any designated reviewer is able to log on, select a review article from this queue, and begin relevance testing. Reviewers have the option to pass the review on to the quality assessment stage or reject the review (i.e., assess it as not relevant). Once a review has passed the relevance stage, it moves to the queue for "articles requiring quality assessment 1," where any reviewer is able to log on and conduct the first quality assessment. The review then moves to a queue for "articles requiring quality assessment 2," where any reviewer, aside from the reviewer who completed quality assessment 1, is able to independently conduct quality assessment 2. All reviews that receive the same quality assessment rating from each independent reviewer move to a holding queue, where the project manager is able to conduct a final check for completeness, then post the article to the live, publicly accessible registry. Articles that receive differing quality assessment ratings from the two independent reviewers are flagged for re-evaluation. Each reviewer receives an e-mail from the system, notifying them that an article they reviewed needs to be reassessed. The two independent reviewers then log on and view their quality assessment tools in a side-by-side view to compare the discrepancies between reviewer ratings. Discrepancies are resolved through consensus. Once the quality assessment ratings are in agreement, the article moves to the holding queue to be posted to the live site and added to the publicly searchable registry.

Creating Health-evidence.ca: Results

As of October 2008, there were 1,364 reviews in the health-evidence.ca registry in 21 public health and health promotion topic areas. Of these, 77% have been assessed as being of strong or moderate methodological quality, with 52% (708) rated as methodologically strong, and 25% (344) as moderate. The 21 topic areas include addiction/substance use, adolescent health, adult health, child health, chronic diseases, communicable disease/infection, dental health, environmental health, food safety and inspection, healthy communities, infant health, injury prevention/safety, mental health, nutrition, parenting, infants and children, physical activity, reproductive health, senior health, sexual health, sexually transmitted infections, and social determinants of health. The most frequently accessed topics include chronic disease prevention, which has 441 reviews, 226 of which are rated as strong; child health, which has 189 reviews, 138 of which are rated as strong; and nutrition, which has 256 reviews, 141 of which are rated as strong.

Since its launch, health-evidence.ca has attracted 3,550 registered users coming from multiple countries, backgrounds, and interests. Approximately 80% of users are Canadian, with most of the remaining 20% from the United States, followed by users from Australia and the U.K. Within Canada, all provinces and territories are represented in the group of registered users, with the largest provinces having the greatest number of users—Ontario, Alberta, and British Columbia—with the fewest users coming from more sparsely populated regions. Public health nurses, program managers, health promotion workers, researchers, and program coordinators are among the largest groups of registered users, followed by librarians, dieticians, medical officers of health, and nutritionists. The majority of users (67%) access the Web site from direct traffic (i.e., have the health-evidence.ca Web page bookmarked, or type it directly into their browser), 20% of users link to health-evidence.ca from a referring site, and 12.5% of users link from a search engine.

In total, health-evidence.ca receives approximately 55,000 visits per year, 30,000 of which are unique visitors. This represents approximately 150 visits per day. Thirty percent of visitors return for multiple visits each year. The average user spends nine minutes on the site and visits five pages per visit. Since the launch of health-evidence.ca, feedback from users has generally been very positive; for example, quotes from users have included "There seems to be something for everyone—I liked that it provides a quality rating for the research—this is something I struggle with—and it holds only what is relevant for us in public health. I will use it as a solid reference point for our programming" (public health manager); "Great!! Your work is of invaluable help for all of us. Thanks very much indeed from Italy" (researcher).

Newsletters are disseminated quarterly to individual users, as well as those who belong to other networks with which health-evidence.ca is partnered. Electronic dissemination of the newsletter coincides with completion of the quarterly updates, where new reviews have been added to the site. This electronic newsletter summarizes the new content posted to health-evidence.ca, as well as categorizes links to reviews assessed as being of strong or moderate methodological quality, according to the twenty-one broad topic areas. This facilitates easier access to relevant evidence for any given user. Monitoring of usage statistics over the past year indicates that significant increases in site visits occur immediately following the release of the electronic newsletter. For example, the release of the March 2008 newsletter resulted in more than 500 site visits daily in the two weeks following release of the newsletter, in comparison to the annual average daily site visit rate of 150. Similar trends were observed following the release of all newsletters in 2008. These user statistics identify health-evidence.ca as an established key resource for public health and health promotion decision makers in Canada and worldwide. While these statistics do not allow inference concerning the incorporation of this evidence into public health policy and practice decisions, the fact that many users return to the site multiple times each year suggests that this KM system is fulfilling a need identified among this target population. In addition, it also is worth noting that the most highly accessed reviews on health-evidence.ca coincide with some of the most pressing policy and practice issues faced by public health decision makers at all levels, from frontline practitioners to senior policymakers. It is encouraging, therefore, that this evidence is being widely accessed during a time when significant policy and practice decisions are being made in these topic areas. The final section of this chapter will provide one example of how the health-evidence.ca KM system was leveraged to quickly, and with minimal resources, address a key need identified by a provincial group of medical officers of health in Canada.

Leveraging a Knowledge Management System for Evidence-Informed Decision Making

Every year the medical officers of health (MOHs) of the thirty-six local public health units in Ontario, Canada, meet on a biannual basis to network and discuss issues of interest. At a meeting of MOHs from the central and central east regions of Ontario in July 2008, consensus was reached about their need for quick-and-easy access to the best available evidence on chronic disease prevention to contribute to upcoming program planning discussions at the local level for the 2009–10 fiscal year. At that time, MOHs identified that while the new Provincial Standards and Programs, set for release during the fall of 2008, would contribute to their program planning decisions, additional evidence would be required with respect to specific interventions and strategies that should be implemented. As a result, the MOHs made a request to the Public Health National Collaborating Centre for Methods and Tools (NCCMT) to assemble the best available evidence in chronic disease prevention.

The mission and mandate of the NCCMT is to enhance evidence-informed public health policy and practice in Canada by improving access to and use of evidence-based methods and tools for stakeholders involved in policymaking, program decision making, practice, and research in Canada. Therefore, this request aligned closely with the NCCMT's mission and mandate, and was only one of many such requests it and health-evidence.ca had received for this type of evidence. A decision was made to explore options for fulfilling this request, with timing being a key issue, since it was July and this evidence was needed for September/October 2008.

The NCCMT, an important partner and funder of health-evidence.ca, met with the health-evidence.ca staff to explore avenues for collaboration and avoid duplication of efforts to fulfill these types of requests. One staff member each from the NCCMT and health-evidence.ca was assigned to work collaboratively on this project and to have a product ready for dissemination within two months. The first step involved the refinement of the research question to clearly identify the population(s), intervention(s), and outcomes of interest. The research question was, "What is the effectiveness of interventions/strategies/policies in preventing chronic diseases across the lifespan?" Health-evidence.ca was then searched, and all reviews evaluating the effectiveness of chronic disease prevention interventions identified (n = 441). Only those reviews (n = 326) identified as being of strong and moderate methodological quality were maintained for future dissemination to public health decision makers. Given there existed such a large number of reviews focused on chronic disease prevention, the reviews were categorized into four major theme areas so as to facilitate searching of this evidence by public health decision makers. The reviews were categorized by disease, population (e.g., children, adults), intervention location (e.g., school, worksite, community), and intervention strategy (e.g., media campaign, support group). Individualized strategies were developed to search health-evidence.ca in real time in each of the four major categories. The value added of developing an internal search mechanism is that it makes it that much easier for decision makers to access the reviews by having to click on just one link (disease, population, setting, and strategy). In addition, given new reviews are added to health-evidence.ca on a quarterly basis, this approach facilitates access to the most up-to-date reviews at all times.

Once the reviews were all categorized and the internal search mechanisms were developed, a communication strategy was created to disseminate the links to the target populations (medical officers of health, public health managers, etc.). First, a one-page communiqué was developed to send electronically to all registered users of health-evidence.ca, as well as the list of contacts and networks health-evidence.ca is affiliated with. This same communiqué also was disseminated to a vast array of decision makers, organizations, and networks known to the NCCMT. The communiqué described why this evidence was compiled, who compiled it, where it was located, and how it could be used to facilitate public health decision making. A shorter version of this communiqué was created in hard copy for distribution at upcoming conferences and meetings. A notice of this resource was inserted on the home page of both health-evidence.ca and the NCCMT, with a link provided to take users directly to the list of the four major theme areas. Users then click on the preferred theme area and are taken to the list of corresponding reviews located on the health-evidence.ca Web site. Therefore, those who access this resource through the NCCMT Web site are transferred directly to the appropriate page on health-evidence.ca, where the searches can be conducted by clicking on the relevant link. Finally, all communication materials were prepared in both English and French. The communication strategy was implemented in early October 2008, meaning the time from initial request for this evidence by the medical officers of health to the provision of these resources to this audience was approximately eight weeks.

While it is difficult to assess at this early stage (three weeks post) the actual impact that the chronic disease resource on health-evidence.ca has had on public health policy and practice, it is possible to provide some statistics with respect to the success of the communication campaign. For example, a notice of release of this chronic disease resource was included in an e-mail distributed to registered users of health-evidence.ca announcing a quarterly update of the health-evidence.ca registry with the addition of 169 new reviews. This e-mail campaign was sent to 2,915 registered users on October 7, 2008. Within one week following distribution of this campaign, statistics metrics indicated that 32% (885) of recipients had opened this e-mail, and 53% (470) of those who opened it had clicked a link; 37 (8%) of the recipients who clicked a link accessed the new chronic disease prevention resource page. Furthermore, a targeted health-evidence.ca e-mail campaign was sent to 3,268 recipients on Friday, October 10, 2008, announcing the launch of the new resource. Those targeted for this communication worked specifically in public health in chronic disease prevention. Within the first week following distribution of this campaign, statistics metrics indicated that 27% (818) of recipients opened this e-mail, and 31% (255) of those who opened it have clicked a link to use the new resource.

Finally, within the first week following the release of the communication material by health-evidence.ca, the chronic disease resource page was the third-ranked viewed page on health-evidence.ca (approximately 500 page views). With respect to the four major theme areas, users accessed the searches by specific diseases most often (386 page views), followed by intervention strategies (305 page views), intervention setting (236 page views), and population (213 page views). Users spent on average forty minutes on the disease specific and intervention strategies pages, thirty-three minutes on intervention setting, and just under one hour on the population page. Announcement of release of this chronic disease resource corresponded to spikes in site visits. On average, health-evidence.ca receives approximately 150 visits per day. In the days following release of this resource, site visits spiked to 1,029 (October 7, 2008), 636 (October 8, 2008), 286 (October 9, 2008), 285 (October 10, 2008), and 286 (October 14, 2008).

Some interesting observations can be made based on these user statistics. The data suggest that, first, there is a high demand for summarized chronic disease prevention evidence; second, public health decision makers respond positively to receiving links to synthesized evidence, as demonstrated by significant increases in site usage when notices of new materials are pushed out to target users; and third, that a tailored campaign, meaning sending topic-relevant materials directly to decision makers, results in much higher rates of accessing the evidence than a more general communication strategy. While further evaluation is needed to test these hypothesizes, these findings provide strong direction with respect to the use of communication strategies for health-evidence.ca in the short term. Furthermore, while these usage statistics are promising and likely indicative of some degree of success, additional research is needed to determine if successful transfer of research evidence to decision makers results in the implementation of public health policies and practice that reflect this evidence.

While the future of health-evidence.ca is dependent on the attainment of funding from relevant public health organizations, the evidence suggests that health-evidence.ca is achieving its goal of facilitating access to high-quality research evidence, so as to promote evidence-informed public health practice. That being said, there is always room for improvement and expansion. For example, the following are some ideas for future site development for health-evidence.ca:

■ Building networks among public health colleagues through a discussion group or groups that can be used as a forum to connect decision makers. Making these links will help decision makers to share ideas and also avoid duplication of work. Live chats are another possible addition to link colleagues (and link colleagues with experts) across the country.

■ Establishing an online discussion group so that users can meet, ask, and answer questions, and network. Discussions will be moderated to ensure appropriate content.

■ Offering online tutorials and case studies that will encourage users to learn more about critically appraising research, interpreting research results, and integrating research into decision making and practice.

In the meantime, as health-evidence.ca turns its attention toward its five-to-ten-year long-term goals, efforts to evaluate the impact of health-evidence.ca are under way, through informal mechanisms, such as the feedback loop within the site, as well as through more rigorous, scientific approaches.

References

1. Lavis, J.N., D. Robertson, J. Woodside, C. McLeod, and J. Abelson. 2003. How can research organizations more effectively transfer research knowledge to decision makers? *The Milbank Quarterly* 81(2):221–48.
2. Lomas, J., T. Culyer, C. McCutcheon, L. McAuley, and S. Law. 2005. Conceptualizing and combining evidence for health system guidance: Final report. Canadian Health Services Research Foundation.
3. Brownson, R.C., J.G. Gurney, and G.H. Land. 1999. Evidence-based decision making in public health. *Journal of Public Health Management and Practice* 5(5):86–97.
4. National Forum on Health. 1998. Canada Health Action: Building on the legacy. Sainte-Foy, Quebec. Editions MultiMondes. Vol. 5.
5. LaPelle, N.R., R. Luckmann, E. Hatheway Simpson, E.R. Martin. 2006. Identifying strategies to improve access to credible and relevant information for public health professionals: A qualitative study. *BMC Public Health* 6:89–101.
6. Dobbins, M., K. DeCorby, P. Robeson, D. Ciliska, H. Thomas, S. Hannah, et al. Feb. 12, 2007. The power of tailored messaging: Preliminary results from Canada's first trial of knowledge brokering. The 5th Canadian Cochrane Symposium: Knowledge for Health.
7. Davis, D.A., M.A. Thomson, A.D. Oxman, and R.B. Haynes. 1992. Evidence for the effectiveness of CME: A review of 50 randomized controlled trials. *Journal of the American Medical Association* 268(9):1111–17.
8. Dobbins, M., B. Davies, E. Danseco, N. Edwards, and T. Virani. 2005. Changing nursing practice: Evaluating the usefulness of a best-practice guideline implementation toolkit. *Nursing Leadership* 18(1):34–48.
9. Lavis, J., H. Davies, A. Oxman, J.L. Denis, K. Golden-Biddle, and E. Ferlie. 2005. Towards systematic reviews that inform health care management and policy-making. *Journal of Health Services Research & Policy* 10(3 Suppl. 1):35–48.
10. Armstrong, R., E. Waters, H. Roberts, S. Oliver, and J. Popay. 2006. The role and theoretical evolution of knowledge translation and exchange in public health. 28(4):384–89.
11. Kelly, M.P., V. Speller, and J. Meyrick. 2004. Getting evidence into practice in public health. NHS Health Development Agency.
12. World Health Organization. 2006. Bridging the "know-do" gap in global health. Accessed Oct. 16, 2008. Available from http://www.who.int/kms/en/.

13. Scarborough, H., J. Swan, and J. Preston. 1999. *Knowledge Management: A Literature Review*. London: Institute of Personnel and Development.
14. Nutley, S., H. Davies, and I. Walter. 2004. *Learning from Knowledge Management: Conceptual Synthesis 2*. University of St. Andrews: Research Unit for Research Utilisation.
15. Stankosky, M. 2005. *Creating the Discipline of Knowledge Management*. Burlington, USA: Elsevier Inc.
16. Knowledge Management. 2008. What is knowledge management? Cited Oct. 16, 2008. Available from http://www.kmhelpdesk.com/.
17. Alavi, M., and D.E. Leidner. 2001. Review: Knowledge management and knowledge management systems: Conceptual foundations and research issues. *MIS Quarterly* 25(1):107–36.
18. Gamble, P.R., and J. Blackwell. 2001. *Knowledge Management: A State of the Art Guide*. London: Kogan Page.
19. Grimshaw, J., M. Eccles, R. Thomas, G. MacLennan, C. Ramsay, C. Fraser, et al. 2006. Toward evidence-based quality improvement: Evidence (and its limitations) of the effectiveness of guideline dissemination and implementation strategies 1966-1998. *Journal of General Internal Medicine* 21(Supplement 2):S14–20.
20. Davis, D., M.A.T. O'Brien, N. Freemantle, F.M. Wolf, P. Mazmanian, and A. Taylor-Vaisey. 1999. Impact of formal continuing medical education: Do conferences, workshops, rounds, and other traditional continuing education activities change physician behavior or health care outcomes? *Journal of the American Medical Association* 282(9):867–74.
21. O'Brien, M.A., S. Rogers, G. Jamtvedt, A.D. Oxman, J.J. Odgaard, D.T. Kristoffersen, et al. 2007. Educational outreach visits: Effects on professional practice and health care outcomes. *Cochrane Database of Systematic Reviews* Issue 4. DOI: 101002/14651858. CD000409. pub2.
22. Ciliska, D., S. Hayward, J. Underwood, and M. Dobbins. 1999. Transferring public health nursing research to health system planning: Assessing the relevance and accessibility of systematic overviews. *Canadian Journal of Nursing Research* 31(1):23–36.
23. Hunt, J.M. 1996. Barriers to research utilization. *Journal of Advanced Nursing* 23:423–25.
24. Shaperman, J. 1995. The role of knowledge utilization in adopting innovation from academic medical centers. *Hospitals & Health Services Administration* 40(3):401–13.
25. Raudonis, B., and H. Griffith. 1991. Model for integrating health services research and health care policy formation. *Nursing & Health Care* 12(1):32–36.
26. Pettengill, M.M., D.A. Gillies, and C.C. Clark. 1994. Factors encouraging and discouraging the use of nursing research findings. *Image: Journal of Nursing Scholarship* 26(2):143–47.
27. Forsetlund, L., and A. Bjorndal. 2002. Identifying barriers to the use of research faced by public health physicians in Norway and developing an intervention to reduce them. *Journal of Health Services Research and Policy* 7(1):10–18.
28. Innvaer, S., G. Vist, M. Trommald, and A. Oxman. 2002. Health policy-makers' perceptions of their use of evidence: A systematic review. *Journal of Health Services Research and Policy* 7(4):239–44.
29. Lee, R.G., and T. Garvin. Feb. 2003. Moving from information transfer to information exchange in health and health care. *Social Science & Medicine* 56(3):449–64.

30. Canadian Health Services Research Foundation. 2004. Is research working for you? Cited March 3, 2007. Available from www.chsrf.ca/other_documents/working_e.php.

31. Fischer, F. 2004. Citizens and experts in risk assessment: Technical knowledge in practical deliberation. *Technology Assessment: Theory and Practice* 13(2):90–98.

32. MacRae, D. 1999. Cross-national perspectives for aiding policy choice. *Journal of Comparative Policy Analysis: Research and Practice* 1:23–37.

33. Dobbins, M., K. DeCorby, and T. Twiddy. 2004. A knowledge transfer strategy for public health decision makers. *Worldviews on Evidence-Based Nursing* 1(2):120–28.

34. Walshe, K., and T.G. Rundall. 2001. Evidence-based management: From theory to practice in health care. *The Milbank Quarterly* 79(3):429–57.

35. Choi, B.C.K., T. Pang, V. Lin, P. Puska, G. Sherman, M. Goddard, et al. 2005. Can scientists and policy makers work together? *Journal of Epidemiology and Community Health* 59(8):632–37.

36. Lomas, J. 2000. Connecting research and policy. ISUMA Spring:140–44.

37. Grol, R., and J. Grimshaw. 2003. From best evidence to best practice: Effective implementation of change in patients' care. *Lancet* 362(9391):1225–30.

38. Lavis, J.N. 1999. Towards a new research transfer strategy for the Institute for Work and Health. Toronto: Institute for Work and Health.

39. Lomas, J., M.A. Enkin, G.A. Anderson, W.J. Hannah, and J. Singer. 1991. Opinion leaders vs audit and feedback to implement practice guidelines: Delivery after previous cesarean section. *Journal of the American Medical Association* 265(17):2202–07.

40. Oxman, A.D., M.A. Thomson, D.A. Davis, and J.E. Hayes. 1995. No magic bullets: A systematic review of 102 trials of interventions to improve professional practice. *Canadian Medical Association Journal* 153(10):1423–31.

41. Kothari, A., S. Birch, and C. Charles. 2005. Interaction and research utilisation in health policies and programs: Does it work? *Health Policy* 71(1):117–25.

42. Battista, R.N. 1989. Innovation and diffusion of health-related technologies. A conceptual framework. *International Journal of Technology Assessment in Health Care* 5(2):227–48.

43. Kaluzny, A.D. 1974. Innovation in health services: Theoretical framework and review of research. *Health Services Research* 9:101–20.

44. McCaughan, D., C. Thompson, N. Cullum, T.A. Sheldon, and D.R. Thompson. 2002. Acute care nurses' perceptions of barriers to using research information in clinical decision-making. *Journal of Advanced Nursing* 39:46–60.

45. Kitson, A., L.B. Ahmed, G. Harvey, K. Seers, and D.R.R. Thompson. 2006. From research to practice: One organizational model for promoting research-based practice. *Journal of Advanced Nursing* 23:430–40.

46. Muir Gray, J.A. 1997. *Evidence-Based Healthcare: How to Make Health Policy and Management Decisions.* Churchill Livingstone, Edinburgh.

47. Funk, S.G., E.M. Tornquist, and M.T. Champagne. 1995. Barriers and facilitators of research utilization. An integrative review. *Nursing Clinics of North America* 30(3):395–407.

48. Kimberly, J.R., and M.J. Evanisko. 1981. Organizational innovation: The influence of individual, organizational, and contextual factors on hospital adoption of technological and administrative innovations. *Academy of Management Journal* 24:689–713.

49. Walczak, J.R., D.B. McGuire, M.E. Haisfield, and A. Beezley. 1994. A survey of research-related activities and perceived barriers to research utilization among professional oncology nurses. *Oncology Nursing Forum* 21:710–15.

50. Nutley, S., I. Walter, and H. Davies. 2002. From knowing to doing: A framework for understanding the evidence-into-practice agenda. University of St. Andrews.

51. Edwards, N., D. Lockett, G. Gurd, and L. Leonard L. 2000. Effectiveness of internet-based dissemination of best practices for public health professionals. Ottawa, Ontario: University of Ottawa.

52. McCartney, P. 1998. The new networking. *American Journal of Maternal/Child Nursing* 23:159–60.

53. Song, S. 1999. Guidelines on the use of electronic networking to facilitate regional or global research networks.

54. Conn, V.S., and J.M. Armer. 1996. Meta-analysis and public policy: Opportunity for nursing impact. *Nursing Outlook* 44(6):267–71.

55. Rychetnik, L., and M. Frommer. 2002. A schema for evaluating evidence on public health interventions. Version 4. National Public Health Partnership, Melbourne.

56. Last, J.M. 1995. *A Dictionary of Epidemiology*. 3rd ed. Oxford University Press.

57. Cook, D.J., C.D. Mulrow, and R.B. Haynes. 1997. Systematic reviews: Synthesis of best evidence for clinical decisions. *Annals of Internal Medicine* 126:376–80.

58. Sandelowski, M., and J. Barroso. 2003. Toward a metasynthesis of qualitative findings on motherhood in HIV-positive women. *Research in Nursing & Health* 26(2):153–70.

59. Jensen, L.A., and M.N. Allen. 1996. Meta-synthesis of qualitative findings. *Qualitative Health Research* 6(4):553–60.

60. Fineout-Overholt, E., D.P. O'Mathuna, and B. Kent. 2008. How systematic reviews can foster evidence-based clinical decisions. *Worldviews on Evidence-Based Nursing* 5(1):45–8.

61. McAuley, L., B. Pham, P. Tugwell, and D. Moher. 2000. Does the inclusion of grey literature influence estimates of intervention effectiveness reported in meta-analyses? *Lancet* 356:1228–31.

62. Ciliska, D., M. Dobbins, and H. Thomas. 2007. Using systematic reviews in health services. In *Reviewing Research Evidence for Nursing Practice: Systematic Reviews*. Webb, C., and B. Roe, eds., 245–53. United States: Wiley-Blackwell, Malden, MA.

63. Ciliska D., A. DiCenso, and G. Guyatt. 2005. Summarizing the evidence through systematic reviews. In *Evidence-Based Nursing: A Guide to Clinical Practice*. DiCenso, A., G. Guyatt, and D. Ciliska, eds., 137–53. St. Louis, Mo.: Elsevier Mosby.

64. Dobbins, M., R. Cockerill, and J. Barnsley. 2001. Factors affecting the utilization of systematic reviews. *International Journal of Technology Assessment in Health Care* 17(2):203–14.

65. Dobbins, M., R. Cockerill, J. Barnsley, and D. Ciliska. 2001. Factors of the innovation, organization, environment, and individual that predict the influence five systematic reviews had on public health decisions. *International Journal of Technology Assessment in Health Care* 17(4):467–78.

66. Dobbins, M., D. Ciliska, R. Cockerill, J. Barnsley, and A. DiCenso. 2002. A framework for the dissemination and utilization of research for health-care policy and practice. *The Online Journal of Knowledge Synthesis for Nursing* 9(7), 149–160.

67. Davies, P. Oct. 24, 2006. Scoping the challenge: Addressing the issues of knowledge transfer and exchange. Keynote address, Canadian Health Services Research Foundation, National Forum on Knowledge Transfer and Exchange.

68. Thomas, H., D. Ciliska, M. Dobbins, and S. Micucci. 2004. A process for systematically reviewing the literature: Providing the research evidence for public health nursing interventions. *Worldviews on Evidence-Based Nursing* 1(3):176–84.

Chapter 10

myPublicHealth

Utilizing Knowledge Management to Improve Public Health Practice and Decision Making

Debra Revere, Paul F. Bugni, Liz Dahlstrom, and Sherrilynne S. Fuller

> Knowledge is of two kinds. We know a subject ourselves, or we know where we can find information upon it.
>
> **Samuel Johnson**, quoted in Boswell's *Life of Johnson*
> English author, critic, and lexicographer (1709–84)

Contents

Introduction

Consider the following scenario:

The local public health department receives a report of three cases of tuberculosis (TB) diagnosed over a one-week time span among a group of homeless men who regularly seek temporary housing at a local urban shelter. Public health professionals have met to discuss the situation and are considering implementing a mandatory symptom screening and skin-test program at all homeless shelters. Before this decision is made they want to know:

- What is the TB case rate among the homeless population?
- What is the number of homeless persons in our city, and what percentage use temporary housing?
- How is a positive tuberculin skin-test result defined?
- What TB treatment and prevention approaches and programs have been most successful in the homeless population?
- What are the legal mandates for reporting? What forms are used, and who is called? What are the local health jurisdiction regulations for reporting?
- Do we have a comprehensive program for the prevention, treatment, and control of TB?
- What is our surge capacity?

The situation above is hypothetical but represents a potentially real reportable disease case faced daily by public health practitioners. Every day, public health professionals at all levels encounter scenarios that require specific information to aid in their day-to-day decision making (Rambo and Dunham, 2000). In public health, timeliness is a key concern, decisions cannot be delayed, and practitioners must be as well-informed as possible. Complicating the situation is the fact that public health is an "umbrella" under which there are many disciplines. Consequently, the public health workforce is diverse, job functions are variable, and often a single individual performs a variety of roles in a public health setting. This diversity of disciplines, backgrounds, and roles presents a challenge to those who are trying to find creative knowledge management solutions that can both broadly and with specificity answer the following public health questions:

- What are the information needs of public health?
- What information sources are most important for meeting these information needs?
- How can access to information be improved and barriers be reduced?
- How can this information be delivered to the right person at the right time and place for it to be used for decision making?
- How can we ensure security of sensitive information?

According to McInerney (2002), "Knowledge management is an effort to increase useful knowledge within the organization. Ways to do this include encouraging communication, offering opportunities to learn, and promoting the sharing of appropriate knowledge artifacts." Knowledge management provides a set of principles and tools to optimize and integrate the processes of creating, sharing, and using knowledge with the goal of creating value for an organization and its community. This chapter reviews the knowledge management approach undertaken to develop myPublicHealth, a customizable content management tool for public health professionals. We describe the project methodology, design process, piloting experiences, and continuing and future developments—all of which incorporate best practices in knowledge management in the development process.

Background

A systematic approach to the development of effective knowledge management systems is critical to public health, and essential for design and implementation of its information and decision support systems. For many years the bulk of research and development on information and decision support systems has focused on the development of integrated clinical decision support systems. This research-and-development push was motivated by the problems identified in maintaining numerous medical information system silos in the 1980s and early 1990s—separate radiology, pharmacy, laboratory systems, etc. This resulted in the integrated environments now utilized in most large medical centers. However, public health practice continues to rely on fragmented information systems which do not provide the real-time decision support capability required to respond to the many population health challenges facing public health today—from epidemics, to environmental disasters, to chronic disease and bioterrorism.

Consider the following respiratory disease scenario:

On Memorial Day weekend, the San Juan Island regional health department is contacted regarding twelve cases of atypical pneumonia with sudden onset of very high fever on Orcas Island (one of the sparsely populated islands of the Pacific Northwest which borders Canada). Access to Orcas is limited to ferry, boats, or small airplanes. Several potential diagnoses are considered, including avian flu, Q fever (*Coxiella burnetii*), SARS, and a possible bioterrorism event. A number of people from China and other parts of the world have been on the island for an international environmental protection meeting, all arriving through the airport in Vancouver, British Columbia. There are rumors that some may have had respiratory illnesses.

The public health nurse called in to this case needs immediate access to risk assessment guidelines, risk management protocols, and environmental and epidemiological information. In addition, she needs to alert health practitioners throughout the islands to anticipate requests for serologic testing and advice regarding containment of the outbreak. While her first impulse is to call the regional epidemiology expert, this individual, along with other key local and state public health officials, are unavailable. The public health nurse confers with the county health officer, who is off the island, and together they hypothesize about the cause of this sudden outbreak in order to make decisions about quarantine and planning next steps until lab tests can be completed. Avian flu seems possible because of the visitors from China and other parts of Asia. What is the current status of Avian flu internationally? However, *C. burnetii* is a possibility as well, since a county fair recently occurred. Could there be a connection between this outbreak and the numerous sheep farms on the islands? Has this happened before? Since the arrest of the terrorist in the nearby city of Port Angeles, bioterrorism is a concern as well. Could there be a weather pattern (e.g., wind shifts) that has contributed to limiting the outbreak so far? What is the probability of an epidemic? Where can the public health nurse and county health officer get this information fast?

In 2001, the President's Information Technology Committee (PITAC) pointed out that the introduction of integrated decision-support systems that can proactively foster best practices requires enhanced information technology methods and tools. Specifically referenced was the need for systems development in support of public health to include "methodologies for automated policy inference that integrate data from diverse sources (e.g., epidemiologic, economic, demographic, geographic), and models of societal resources and values to suggest plausible public health responses to major health problems" (PITAC, 2001). PITAC recommended that the following be undertaken:

- Expand the range and granularity of routinely captured data.
- Standardize terminology.
- Develop robust techniques for incorporating new data types into existing clinical data repositories.
- Organize and collect large-scale databases to determine best practices.
- Develop guidelines based on such evidence.
- Implement guidelines at the point of use, including embedded decision support that is continually updated as new evidence accumulates.
- Reduce the cost and difficulty of integrating applications that reside on heterogeneous technologies.

In October 2005, the University of Washington in Seattle, Washington, was awarded one of the first Centers for Disease Control and Prevention (CDC) grants to establish a Center of Excellence in Public Health Informatics (CEPHI). CEPHI's mission is to improve the public's health through discovery, innovation, and research related to health information and information technology.

As stated, the public health environment is complicated by a diverse workforce, composed of individuals from many domains—including physicians, nurses, and administrators—and environments—local, state, tribal, and national—whose job functions can be at cross-purposes to one another, are overlapping, and have varying information demands. Yet each of the above recommendations can be addressed by implementing a knowledge management approach in the public health environment with the goal of providing a means to deliver the right information to the right person and place at the right time. Knowledge management in the public health context can be used ". . . to capture knowledge needed to ensure public health preparedness, to manage existing information more effectively, and to enable public health professionals to work collaboratively in a virtual environment" (ASTHO, 2005).

The myPublicHealth Project is one of two research projects funded through CEPHI. The goal of myPublicHealth is the design and development of an interactive, customizable, digital knowledge management system to support the collection, management, and retrieval of public health documents, forms, datasets, training materials, "people" resources, and tools. The knowledge management system aims to improve access to and use of digital information resources in support of evidence-based public health practice. The long-term goal is the creation of a comprehensive knowledge management approach that is tailored to the public health practitioner's information needs, work processes, and environment.

Achieving these goals requires a comprehensive understanding of the information needs, information-seeking behavior, and human–computer interaction of public health practitioners. Library and information science research describes information seeking as situational, contextual, and unique to the information seeker. Users experience gaps in knowledge that interfere with their ability to articulate what they know and do not know, and knowledge of users' tasks can help point to systems designed to support those tasks (Hewins, 1990; Wilson, 1994).

Methodology

Prior to system design, we designed a knowledge management methodology for understanding the public health practitioner's information needs, work context, and available resources. The pre-implementation plan included the following tasks: (1) a comprehensive literature review focused on understanding the unique information needs of myPublicHealth users; (2) an inventory of public health information sources cross-referenced by discipline or role (e.g., communicable disease specialist, public health nurse, health educator) and content area (e.g., epidemiology, datasets, animal health); and (3) a workflow analysis to delineate essential functions and information usage regarding the real-life decision support needs of public health practitioners in a variety of settings. From these tasks we developed our initial user and system requirements, which informed prototyping efforts and evaluation approach.

Literature Review of Public Health Workforce Information Needs

Before developing system requirements, we undertook a comprehensive literature review focused on the following questions: (1) What are the information needs of public health professionals? (2) In what ways are those needs currently being met? (3) What are the barriers to meeting those needs? (4) What is the role of the Internet in meeting information needs?

We found that although few formal studies of information needs and information-seeking behaviors of public health professionals have been reported, the literature consistently indicated a critical need for comprehensive, coordinated, and accessible information. The review concluded the following:

1. Selection of public health information resources is influenced by job function, disciplines, and training, as well as experience with incorporating external information resources into work.
2. Public health practitioners meet their information needs by using information resources that are easy to access and use, up to date, flexible, free or low cost, predigested or summarized, stable, and are focused on the practitioners' particular field(s).
3. Given the variety of roles, functions, disciplines, and backgrounds of the workforce, a one-size-fits-all system cannot adequately meet public health worker information needs.
4. Colleagues, peers, program personnel, state contacts, and other people are the most reliable, available, and commonly used information resources for carrying out the day-to-day work of public health.
5. Valued information resources can be described as vetted, high quality, generated by an authoritative content source, verifiable by a trusted source, up to date and known to be regularly updated, convenient, and accessible. (Revere et al., 2007).

The findings indicated that public health needs a customizable public health knowledge management system and user interface with optimal interoperability and the capability to provide timely access with the following features:

1. Reflect the complexity and diversity of the public health workforce itself, for example, with the design of customizable views and customized information "toolkits."
2. Reduce major barriers to information access, including time, resource reliability, trustworthiness and credibility of information, and "information overload" of both relevant and irrelevant information.
3. Offer ready access at the point of need, with a high level of security but easy user access to needed information (e.g., single sign-on access).
4. Include avenues that support timely access to human communication networks (e.g., providing accurate directories, Listservs, etc.).
5. Provide user-friendly interfaces and smart search systems.
6. Support easy addition of locally useful information at the individual and at the department levels.

Based upon this extensive literature review, we concluded that "(n)either the creation nor the distribution of information resources [defined as data, guidelines, research findings, maps, policies, laws, evaluation metrics, teaching material] upon which public health practitioners depend is managed in any systematic or comprehensive way at the present time" (Revere et al., 2007).

Inventory of Public Health Information Sources and Utilization by Roles: Resources Matrix

Building a knowledge management system requires an understanding of the necessary knowledge objects to populate the system. Public health practice encompasses numerous disciplines, and public health practitioners often take on a variety of roles as part of their day-to-day work. A constant stream of information of critical importance is produced at local, state, national, and international levels. In daily decision-making process, public health professionals at all levels encounter the need for specific pieces of information—i.e., disease incidence data (county, state, national), vaccination guidelines, industrial effluent data, laws and regulations, legislative issues updates, metadata on data sets, outcome measurement resources, and synthesized knowledge bases of information and guidelines, among many others (Rambo and Dunham, 2000).

In the event of a disease outbreak or other public health emergency, public health professionals often are reduced to scrambling through piles of paper reports in their offices, searching for the relevant recent report or statistical information that would help them develop an effective response. Relevant resources to support public health decision making span a multiplicity of publication formats (e.g., print and electronic) produced at local, state, national, and international levels. Topic areas can include disease incidence data (county, state, national), vaccination guidelines, industrial effluent data, laws and regulations, legislative issues updates, metadata on data sets, outcome measurement resources, and synthesized knowledge bases of information and guidelines, among others. However, a limited amount of this critical information is published through standard channels, and finding a resource that is targeted to answering a question can be difficult for busy public health professionals.

We inventoried public health information resources identified from public health practitioner interviews, surveys, sources identified in the literature review, and preliminary findings of a workflow assessment at two public health departments. This inventory was collated and cross-referenced into an information resources matrix. Constructing a matrix is a methodology for summarizing a comprehensive specification and relationship between candidate information resources and potential users. The first column in the matrix lists the specific candidate resources utilized by public health. These are divided into two categories: resource content areas (e.g., epidemiology, datasets, animal health) and user roles or discipline (e.g., communicable disease specialist, public health nurse, health educator).

Table 10.1 shows a portion of the original matrix, which contains more than 200 information resources cross-referenced to nine content-area toolkits and five workforce roles. The resources matrix provided the framework for prioritizing and organizing content based on demand.

Table 10.1 Information Resources Matrix (portion)

	Content Toolkit			Workforce Role	
Information Resource	*Zoo*	*Epi*	*EBPH*	*CHS*	*EHS*
AHRQ guide to clinical preventive services			X		
Air quality management					X
ASTHO EBM PH			X		
Epi-Info		X		X	
Canary database, Animals as Sentinels of Human Environmental Health Hazards (Yale)	X				
Cancer registry				X	
CCDM		X			
Community guide (CDC)			X	X	
CDC Division of Parasitic Diseases	X	X		X	X

Information Resource	Content Toolkit			Workforce Role	
	Zoo	Epi	EBPH	CHS	EHS
DARE: Database of Abstracts of Reviews of Effects			X		
DEBI: Diffusion of Effective Behavioral Interventions Database			X	X	
Directory of PH veterinarians by state	X				
DOH Epi trends		X		X	
Emerging infectious diseases		X	X		
Environmental health perspectives					X
Epi-Info		X		X	
E-roadmap to evidence-based PH practice			X		
Guide to community preventive services				X	
H-CUP: Healthcare Cost & Utilization Project		X		X	
HSDB: Hazardous Substances Data Bank		X	X		X
Merck veterinary manual: Global zoonoses table	X				
MMWR		X	X		
NEISS: National Electronic Injury Surveillance System		X		X	
NIOSH pocket guide to chemical hazards					X
Prevention communication research database				X	
ToxNET					X
U.S. Census Bureau		X			
Washington state DOH Division of Environmental Health					X

Source: From Revere and Fuller, 2008.

Note: Zoo = animal health; Epi = epidemiology; EBPH = evidence-based public health; CHS = community health specialist; EHS = environmental health specialist.

Workflow Analysis

A critical but often overlooked step in information system design is to understand the fit of the system into the work environment of the users. Workflow analysis to delineate essential functions and information usage regarding the real-life decision support needs of public health practitioners has been conducted in a variety of settings (e.g., Blaya et al., 2007; Fontanesi et al., 2002; Turner et al., 2008). The research literature on workflow analysis in health systems design indicates that:

1. The complexity and breadth of public health services and tasks, along with a chronic shortage of funds, have prevented the widespread incorporation of information systems at the local level (Turner et al., 2004, 2005).
2. Practitioners are frustrated by lack of integration across bibliographic databases, ready answers to questions (as opposed to lists of references or links to Web sites), and access to data tables and figures within publications which are a primary focus for gathering information for forming hypotheses and answering questions (Fuller et al., 2004; Rambo, 1998; Revere et al., 2004; Revere and Fuller, 2005).
3. Premature adoption of computerized systems that fails to take into consideration user values, needs, and practices and organization issues may have unintended consequences that are costly and unsafe, such as failed systems, inefficient work, and inability to use data (Ash, 2004; Kirah et al., 2005; Markus, 2004).
4. As a new information system goes through its development and implementation stage, an iterative process must take place to integrate the assumptions made by the designers of the system and the people that use them (Forsythe, 1992).

A key methodological component is to incorporate collaborative requirements specifications when considering implementation of an information system in the public health environment—that is, development must incorporate the users in defining system requirements, and developers must understand the business and objectives of public health. By understanding a business process and its multiple components, including triggers, inputs, outputs, and objectives, we begin to understand how an information system, that is, a tool that supports work, must perform to add value to the users. It is known that a number of clinical decision support systems have failed or had reduced usability because this critical step was omitted (Müller et al., 2000; Timpka and Johansson, 1994). Once business processes are defined, one can define in detail the specific things the information system must do—that is, the requirements—to make the process achieve its purpose and be efficient (PHII, 2006). Research on decision support tools indicates that users seek nonintrusive tools available at the point and time of need. In addition, role-based tools—i.e., tools relevant to a specific work role and function, such as the tools a public health nurse prefers to use, as opposed to the tools a community health educator will prefer—are desirable over tools that may or may not be useful to the task at hand (Fuller et al., 1999; Tarczy-Hornoch et al., 1997).

Rapid Prototyping and Iterative Interface Design

Rapid prototyping is a collaborative software engineering method that "enables users to become involved at the design stage, thereby allowing requirements that would have surfaced after deployment of a system to be uncovered early" (Dean et al., 1997). The approach is a cycle in which user evaluation and implementation of the system are in a feedback loop, with the results of testing at each cycle feeding into the design focus of the next cycle (Eliot et al., 2002). In addition, by involving users in the evolution of a project's life cycle, rapid prototyping integrates specialized stakeholder knowledge and iteratively improves understanding of the requirements. Utilizing this approach, we created a prototype system that underwent usability testing for one year by public health stakeholders.

Rather than implement a single proof-of-concept demonstration, we modified the interface and content over several phases during the year. This multiphased prototyping approach allowed us to gather feedback and requirements at different stages of development. The prototyping process was initiated with a group of users using a paper mock-up. Prototyping then moved to an operational online flat HTML prototype with limited content, released to enable iterative design testing and feedback with local health department practitioners. Rapid prototyping was used to translate this feedback into system specifications and interface design of the prototype system. Prior to release of successive versions, an expert review by a small group of faculty and practitioners was conducted to evaluate consistency of the interface design's layout, terminology, color, etc. This group also provided an informal cognitive walkthrough of the site before each release. Based on feedback, the look and feel of the interface was refined, critical resources identified for addition, and some resources were removed. Prototyping also informed finalization of software requirements specifications, software system architecture, and interface design user test plans and procedures. The prototype interface and digital content repository underwent six major revisions. A more detailed explanation of this process can be found in Revere and Fuller, 2008, and Revere et al., 2007b.

As with all other methodological approaches, the design and requirements gathering cycle was informed by knowledge management principles that emphasize the importance of people in any knowledge management endeavor. Building a collective and collaborative user-designer relationship by involving users from the beginning with paper mock-ups and presentations to our target audience, we not only gathered important feedback and suggestions, but built a group of early adopters and promoters for myPublicHealth who would pave the way for its success.

An important outcome of initial prototyping was our understanding that our users wanted flexibility and control over the interface and delivery of the content. Our solution was to use a content management system (CMS), a publishing system that streamlines the process of creating, managing, and delivering content. To accommodate the CMS requirement, we investigated various Web site technologies that would enable us to develop a customizable and easily maintained system. The major decision was whether to use a proprietary software or open-source solution for building myPublicHealth.

System Architecture and Design

Open-source software are free applications released under special licensing terms that allow the core coding to be viewed and edited to suit the needs of the user. Open source has been described as a community-centric development model maintained and supported by a network of individuals who build on the work that has been done by others and encourages the free flow of knowledge and insight between all community members (Kerr, 2007). Given our adherence to knowledge management principles in building myPublicHealth, it was decided that an open-source solution was the most fitting approach to take.*

Several open-source CMSs (Plone, Wikis, Mambo, Alfresco, Drupal, Joomla!) were evaluated for the following capabilities: ease of assembly and configuration, availability of documentation and support, delivery of information, customizability of user interface, integration with existing or desired local systems modules, hosting demands and costs, cross-platform capability, ability to handle multiple document formats, and multiple security level options.

We wanted to build a system that could be used on any platform, had a centralized authentication mechanism, met accessibility guidelines, supported metadata creation, and could link to external data sources. We chose the Plone content management system, which most closely matched our requirements (Plone CMS). In addition, Plone was chosen for its extensibility, supportive open-source developer community, and a flexible workflow model, which allows content or portions of the site to be visible and editable only by its owner and others with appropriate access to the folder in which they reside. This last feature is a requirement in a public health environment in which data may be viewable by individuals with a specific level of permission or in a specific role. In April 2007, we implemented a beta version of myPublicHealth, using as its infrastructure the Plone CMS.

---

* Details regarding the advantages and disadvantages of open source, as well as the philosophical and ethical rationale often used to promote open source, are beyond the scope of this chapter and can be found in Fitzgerald, 2006; Kerr, 2007; and Von Hippel, 2001.

Collaborative Tool Development

As stated previously, partnering with stakeholders has been the primary approach used in our collaborative design process, and iterative designing represents a knowledge management approach, as it emphasizes the involvement of the people who will use the system. We continued this partnership with successive releases of myPublicHealth. In order to improve the content, interface, navigability and structure, users entering the site are asked to identify themselves by role(s)—administration, clinical staff (emergency and nonemergency), community health specialist (including evaluation and assessment), emergency responder (including bioterrorism and preparedness), emergency health specialist, environmental health specialist, epidemiologist, training, and veterinary or animal health specialist. Usage data by role is collected and drives the refinement and revision of existing content on the site.

Based on feedback from our users, myPublicHealth includes public health documents, datasets, training materials and tutorials, and tools, as well as content accessible through specialized search boxes. Content is grouped according to five workforce roles and eight resource-based toolkits, in addition to the home page (see Figure 10.1). Resources are organized for search and presentation using current metadata standards, and are accessible through the Web-based interface: tabs across the top of the interface (A) provide access to toolkits populated with information content organized by public health content areas. Resources organized by public health roles (B) can be selected from a suite of resources accessed from the left navigation bar. Specialized searching services (C) are accessible through the numerous search boxes for querying directly into resources. Figure 10.2 is a screen shot of one of the role-based pages, the epidemiology page.

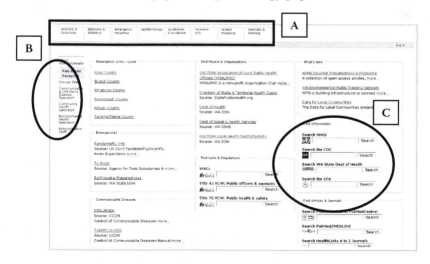

Figure 10.1   myPublicHealth home page, http://myph.org, Version 8.03.3.

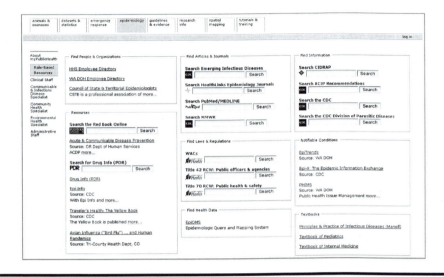

Figure 10.2   myPublicHealth epidemiology page, http://myph.org/epidemiology.

User feedback and usage statistics continue to inform both content and layout of the site and led to incorporating additional public health practice utilities and technologies, such as data sources and specialized mapping tools. Users have reported that the myPublicHealth interface, content, search, and navigational tools "...fits their mental model of a how a system in public health should support information seeking." Particularly popular features are the search boxes that utilize specialized Google domain searches of key Web sites, including the CDC, World Health Organization, and the Washington state legislative and administrative codes. In addition, users report that the role-based access approach, which allows them to quickly drill into work-function-based information, is highly useful. The Washington state system is being used at all levels of service—local, statewide, rural, tribal, and urban—for public health agencies to retrieve evidence-based information needed for public health decision support.

Enhancing Interoperability

Interoperability across resources in a knowledge repository is a way for users to search, discover, access, and retrieve needed information. This can be achieved by applying a consistent and structured metadata schema, which identifies the elements needed to describe a resource in a standardized way to its contents. However, unlike the fields of clinical medicine or genomics, the diversity of the field of public health has challenged efforts to standardize public health terminology (Humphreys et al., 1997). myPublicHealth uses an expanded and customized vocabulary schemata based on the Unified Medical Language System (McCray et al., 1996) by incorporating a standard metadata structure of descriptive, technical, structural, and administrative descriptors as the basis for management and discovery of the myPublicHealth knowledge repository's digital assets.

While the myPublicHealth ontology is still in development at the time of writing this chapter, this metadata core standard also will be the schema through which commonalities and mappings are established for sharing information about existing, distributed resources. In addition, we are adhering to the Public Health Information Network Messaging System (PHINMS) vocabulary standards and specifications. Developed by the CDC and national partners, PHINMS is a key component in supporting the development and deployment of standards-based public health information systems: "PHIN Vocabulary Standards and Specifications seek to promote the use of standards-based vocabulary within PHIN systems and foster the use and exchange of consistent information among public health partners. The use of PHIN Vocabulary Standards and Specifications ensures that vocabularies are aligned . . . for authoring, mapping, editing and distributing standards-based vocabularies to local, state and national PHIN partners" (PHINMS).

Next Steps

As stated previously, understanding the information needs of public health is a first step in building a knowledge management tool that can provide the right information to the right person in the right place and time to support decision making. Building, testing, and iteratively rebuilding a tool in a knowledge management collaboration with users was the next step. However, public health practitioners need tools that can be tailored to their individual needs, whether they are a state health department-level epidemiologist who has overall responsibility for state disease surveillance activities or a public health nurse in a small, rural health jurisdiction who wears multiple hats in providing direct care and health promotion services for individuals, families, and community groups. Providing a way for users to customize myPublicHealth, perhaps by expanding the capabilities of the tool so users could set up their own personal Web pages or individual departments or divisions within a public health jurisdiction could customize their toolkits to include the resources most germane to their work functions, was the next step.

Piloting an Embedded Knowledge Management System in a Public Health Setting: myPublicHealth Montana

The long-term goal of myPublicHealth is the implementation of a successful knowledge management system that is tailored to the public health practitioner's information needs, work processes, and environment. Assessing the procedural feasibility and advantages of utilizing a *customizable* decision-making tool for public health practitioners requires more than monitoring Web site traffic through usage logs. To test whether users would customize the interface and content suite, a pilot project was launched in February 2008 in collaboration with the Montana State Department of Health and Human Services (DPHHS). Our question: Would public health practitioners tailor myPublicHealth to the unique regional needs of the Montana public health workforce and use it to manage the collection, description, management, and retrieval of evidence-based information needed for public health decision making?

Prior to launching the pilot, and to inform our content and customization protocols, we conducted the following activities to better understand the Montana public health environment and information needs and to engage our pilot stakeholders:

1. A pre-implementation questionnaire asking respondents for background demographics (age, education, job title, years in current position, etc.), current resource use, technical expertise, list of browser bookmarks, and problems experienced when practicing public health was circulated. Response rate was eighty-four percent and enabled us to build a resource matrix (as seen in Table 10.1) specific to Montana users.
2. Phone interviews were conducted with all DPHHS bureau chiefs, asking questions about resource use, barriers to accessing resources, and information needs. We also asked bureau chiefs to describe the latest problem experienced during the work day that led to an interruption in routine or made work less effective in order to create a use-case scenario for myPublicHealth.
3. Staff traveled to Helena, Mont., to visit the DPHHS facilities and meet with bureau chiefs, public health practitioners, and information technology and staff members. This visit included introducing the concept of myPublicHealth to public health practitioners and providing a series of training sessions to designated content managers on using the CMS software. In addition, we provided training on improving online search skills, finding "hard-to-find" public health resources, and information management.

Responses to interviews and the questionnaire built a "snapshot" of resources (online, hard copy, and "people") used with greatest frequency, knowledge of public health resources, and how our users organize needed information. Visiting Montana further informed our understanding of the barriers public health practitioners encounter in accessing needed information and the limitations in their technical infrastructure and support.

In April 2008, we rolled out the first version of http://mt.myph.org with an expansion and enhancement of existing myPublicHealth resources tailored to the state of Montana. At the time of writing this chapter, content managers are collaborating with the myPublicHealth knowledge management group to modify the look and feel of mt.myph.org to conform to regional preferences. Initially, Montana opted to organize the interface according to bureau-based toolkits—chronic disease prevention, health promotion, communicable disease control and prevention, family and community health, health planning, laboratory services, preparedness, and environmental health—as opposed to the role- or content-based resources organization of the Washington state myPublicHealth. However, after the generic interface changed, we discovered that usage dropped and users preferred the earlier organization by toolkit and roles. Currently, we are assisting our Montana pilot colleagues in modifying the interface back to its original organizational framework (Revere et al., 2008).

Evaluation of the Montana pilot will include three tasks: (1) research whether and how public health practitioners will adapt and customize myPublicHealth for their own knowledge management purposes; (2) determine what content is most needed by users that will in turn inform continuing design of the customizability and personalization features; and (3) understand how myPublicHealth can be seamlessly incorporated into the users' work environment. At the time of this writing, plans were under way to begin this evaluation in January 2009.

Rather than emphasizing the technical development, we have incorporated a user-collaborative approach in general, and specifically in working with our Montana pilots. "Focusing exclusively on the technical issues of electronic collaboration is a sure way to a very expensive failure. . . . A focus on the people issues dramatically increases the potential for success" (McInerney, 2002). And yet, this same focus on the people side of knowledge management has created its own barriers and issues, especially when—in the case of Montana—the impact of geographic distance on deliberations about content, etc., is added. We will be evaluating whether this approach will reduce time spent searching across and through materials, enhance decision making, and improve the overall quality of public health services.

Conclusion

The goal of a knowledge management endeavor is to create value. Our long-term goal is the implementation of a successful and customizable knowledge management system that is tailored to the public health practitioner's information needs, work processes, and environment, and provides timely access to public health information and resources in support of decision making at the point and time of need. We have utilized a knowledge management approach in emphasizing the creation, capture, sharing, and leveraging of information that is systematically gathered, managed, used, analyzed, and made available for sharing and discovery in a public health organization. By reducing uncertainty, promoting the collective sharing of information with a knowledge repository, codifying knowledge assets so they can be easily found, and engaging stakeholders throughout the process, myPublicHealth ultimately creates value.

Acknowledgments

We wish to acknowledge the contributions of others to the myPublicHealth Project, including Yuki Durham, AnnMarie Kimball, John Kobayashi, Ann Madhavan, Mark Oberle, Svend Sorenson, and Anne Turner. Funding for myPublicHealth is provided by the Centers for Disease Control and Prevention Award Number 1 P01 CD000261-01 (M. Oberle, principal investigator), which supports the Center for Public Health Informatics in the School of Public Health, University of Washington, Seattle, Washington.

References

Ash, J. 2004. Some unintended consequences of information technology in health care: The nature of patient care information system-related errors. *J Am Med Inform Assoc* 11(2):104–12.

ASTHO. 2005. Knowledge management for public health professionals. Available at http://www.astho.org/pubs/ASTHO-Knowledge-Management.pdf.

Blaya, J.A., S.S. Shin, M.J. Yagui, G. Yale, C.Z. Suarez, L.L Asencios, J.P. Cegielski, and H.S. Fraser. 2007. A web-based laboratory information system to improve quality of care of tuberculosis patients in Peru: Functional requirements, implementation and usage statistics. *BMC Med Inform Decis Mak* 7:33.

Centers for Disease Control and Prevention. Public Health Information Network Messaging System. Available at http://www.cdc.gov/phin/software-solutions/phinms/index.html.

Dean, D.L., J.D. Lee, M.O. Pendergast, A.M. Hickey, and J.F. Nunamaker. 1997. Enabling the effective involvement of multiple users: Methods and tools for collaborative software engineering. *J Manage Inform Sys* 14(3):179–222.

Eliot, M., T. Robinson, R. Mayberry, J. Ramey, and B. Stewart. 2002. Rolling assessment: Observing on-going user responses to a Next Generation Internet telemedicine application through successive stages of development. Proc Soc for Tech Commun Annu Conf, 281–5.

Fontanesi, J., M. De Guire, J. Chiang, D. Kopald, K. Holcomb, and M.H. Sawyer. 2002. The forms that bind: Multiple data forms result in internal disaggregation of immunization information. *J Public Health Manag Pract* 8(2):50–5.

Forsythe, D.E. 1992. Using ethnography to build a working system: Rethinking basic design assumptions. Proceedings of the Annual Symposium in Computer Applied Medical Care, 505–9.

Fuller, S.S., D.S. Ketchell, P. Tarczy-Hornoch, and D. Masuda D. 1999. Integrating knowledge resources at the point of care: Opportunities for librarians. *Bull Med Libr Assoc* 87(4):393–403.

Fuller, S.S., D. Revere, P.F. Bugni, and G.M. Martin. 2004. A knowledgebase system to enhance scientific discovery: Telemakus. *Biomed Digit Libr* 1(1):2.

Hewins, E.T. 1990. Information need and use studies. *Ann Rev Info Sci Tech* 25:145–72.

Humphreys, B.L., A.T. McCray, and M.L. Cheh. 1997. Evaluating the coverage of controlled health data terminologies: Report on the results of the NLM/AHCPR large scale vocabulary test. *J Am Med Inform Assoc* 4(6):484–500.

Kirah, A., C. Fuson, J. Grudin, and E. Feldman. 2005. Ethnography for software development. In *Cost Justifying Usability: An Update for the Internet Age.* 2nd ed. Bias, R., and D. Mayhew, eds., 415–45. Elsevier.

Markus, M.L. 2004. Technochange management: Using IT to drive organizational change. *J Inform Tech* 19(1):4–20.

McCray, A.T., A.M. Razi, A.K. Bangalore, A.C. Browne, and P.Z. Stavri. 1996. The UMLS Knowledge Source Server: A versatile Internet-based research tool. Proceedings of AMIA Annual Fall Symposium, 164–8.

McInerney, C. 2002. Knowledge management and the dynamic nature of knowledge. *J Am Soc Info Sci Techn* 53(2):1009–18.

Müller, M.L., T. Ganslandt, H.P. Eich, K. Lang, C. Ohmann, and H.U. Prokosch. 2000. Integrating knowledge based functionality in commercial hospital information systems. *Stud Health Technol Inform* 77:817–21.

PHII. 2006. *Taking Care of Business: A Collaboration to Define Local Health Department Business Processes.* Decatur, Ga.: Public Health Informatics Institute. Available at http://www.phii.org/Files/Taking_Care_of_Business.pdf.

PITAC. 2001. *Transforming Health Care through Information Technology.* Arlington, Va.: National Coordination Office for Information Technology Research and Development.

Plone CMS. Open Source Content Management System. Available at http://plone.org/.

Rambo, N. 1998. Information resources for public health practice. *J Urban Health: Bull New York Acad of Med* 75(4):807–25.

Rambo, N., and P. Dunham. 2000. Information needs and use of the public health workforce—Washington, 1997–1998. *MMWR Morb Mortal Wkly Rep* 49(6):118–20.

Revere, D., and S.S. Fuller. 2005. Characterizing biomedical concept relations: Concept relationships as a pathway for knowledge creation and discovery. In *Medical Informatics: Advances in Knowledge Management and Data Mining in Biomedicine.* Chen, H., S. Fuller, and A. McCray, eds., 183–210. Boston: Kluwer.

Revere, D., and S. Fuller. 2008. Building a customizable knowledge management environment to support public health practice: Design strategies. In Proceedings of Hawaii International Conference on System Sciences, Honolulu, Hawaii.

Revere, D., S. Fuller, P.F. Bugni, and G.M. Martin. 2004. An information extraction and representation system for rapid review of the biomedical literature. *Medinfo* 11(Pt 2):788–92.

Revere, D., A. Turner, A. Madhavan, N. Rambo, P.F. Bugni, A.M. Kimball, and S.S. Fuller. 2007a. Understanding the information needs of public health practitioners: A literature review to inform design of an interactive digital knowledge management system. *J Biomed Informat* (special issue on public health informatics) 40(4):410–21.

Revere, D., P. Bugni, and S.S. Fuller. 2007b. A public health knowledge management repository that includes grey literature. *Grey J* 3(3):164–68.

Revere, D., P. Chilana, S. Helgerson, and S. Fuller. 2008. Building and piloting a customizable knowledge management environment to support public health practice: myPublicHealth. In Proceedings of the MLA Annual Meeting, Chicago.

Tarczy-Hornoch, P., T.S. Kwan-Gett, L. Fouche, J. Hoath, S. Fuller, K.N. Ibrahim, D.S. Ketchell, J.P. LoGerfo, and H.I. Goldberg. 1997. Meeting clinician information needs by integrating access to the medical record and knowledge resources via the Web. In Proceedings of the AMIA Annul Fall Symposium, 7:809–13.

Timpka, T., and M. Johansson. 1994. The need for requirements engineering in the development of clinical decision-support systems: A qualitative study. *Methods Inf Med* 33(2):227–33.

Turner, A.M., E.D. Liddy, J.A. Bradley, J.A. Wheatley, and S.B. Corieri. 2004. Improved access to the public health grey literature through automatically generated document surrogates. *MedInfo* 11(Pt 2):1890.

Turner, A., E.D. Liddy, J. Bradley, J. Wheatly, and S.B. Courieri. 2005. Modeling public health interventions for improved access to the public health gray literature. *J Med Libr Assoc* 93(4):487–94.

Turner, A.M., Z. Stavri, D. Revere, and R. Altamore. From the ground up: Determining the information needs and resources of public health nurses in an Oregon county health department. *J Med Libr Assoc.* In press.

Wilson, T.D. 1994. Information needs and uses: Fifty years of progress. In *Fifty Years of Information Progress: A Journal of Documentation Review*. Vickery, B.C., ed., 15–51. London: Aslib.

Chapter 11

Connections
Sharing Experience to Advance Public Health Practice

Ellen Wild and Debra Bara

If you want to travel fast, go alone. If you want to travel far, go together.
African Proverb

Contents

Introduction

In 1999, Rhoda Nicholas faced a tough challenge. As the newly appointed chief information officer (CIO) at the Utah State Department of Health, her mission was to integrate a wide range of independently functioning information systems that needed to operate as one. At the time, this was a novel approach not only for Utah, but also for information systems in general. Success in this new role was critical to meeting the strategic needs of the agency in improving public health services and health outcomes throughout the state of Utah. Moreover, in the past, the position of CIO did not exist at the department level, and not everyone thought there was a need for one. Rhoda explained, "People were incredulous at the beginning; they wondered why we needed a role like this." She was undertaking a mission that most did not understand, did not buy into, and for which there was no roadmap.

Rhoda began to explore her options for action. She knew what she wanted— to learn from others who were in a similar situation. Her ideas first started taking shape when she participated in an immunization registry meeting in which the Public Health Informatics Institute (the Institute) staff discussed the possibility of creating a community of practice. "I liked the Institute staff; I liked the idea behind the concept—bringing people together to work on a common problem and to learn from each other. I knew something like that would be a good thing to help me achieve success in my new role as CIO."

By participating in the Institute's collaborative process, Rhoda realized that an approach to problem solving that engaged others who were working on the same issues would be helpful. She knew that she would benefit from sharing knowledge, discussing ideas, and learning from colleagues who were spread across the United States, but shared the common goal of building information systems to support the new way health departments were being asked to operate. As one of the first states in the U.S. to undertake development of immunization registries and the integration of child health information systems, Utah was an early adopter of using technology to support improvement in health status of populations. "Being new in the Department of Health, I wanted an opportunity to bounce ideas off of others. I wanted to compare and contrast what everyone else was doing and learn from others as we all progressed. I knew there would be a benefit from hearing about the challenges and successes of my colleagues."

Rhoda noted one of the attributes of communities of practice that she came to value: "Knowledge grows in all directions simultaneously. The sum of that type of knowledge ends up being greater than that which any single one of us could have come up with. We innovate, we don't repeat the same mistakes, and we collaborate on ideas that create something that benefits the whole."

Rhoda did not know it at the time, but she was the impetus for the creation of *Connections*, a community of practice developed by the Institute for public health practitioners working on integrating their early child health information systems. Rhoda's need to learn from others in the same situation prompted the Institute to create what was to become one of the first communities of practice formally established in the public health arena. The Institute realized that the problems Rhoda had faced would soon be experienced by many public health leaders.

When Rhoda began the task of integrating Utah's child health information systems in 1999, she was at the advent of a situation that increasingly affects today's public health workforce: Unprecedented demands are forcing creative responses to address increasingly complex problems. Current challenges in public health include not only tracking and containing emerging infectious diseases, but also responding to emergencies and disasters and preventing chronic diseases. In this information-driven era, public health is asked to provide more information faster and link electronically with partners in the private health care sector. In addition, leaders are concerned about the out migration of knowledge holders—retirement of the experienced members of the public health workforce. In some public health organizations, communities of practice have been recognized as a potential strategy to harness the knowledge of the experienced workforce and assist in achieving organizational goals and objectives. The *Connections* community of practice (CoP) is an example of a community that has shaped the practice of public health informatics.

The Public Health Informatics Institute's Communities of Practice

The Public Health Informatics Institute is a program of the Task Force for Child Survival and Development (the Task Force), an international nonprofit organization. Started in 2000 by David A. Ross, Sc.D., the Institute grew out of a program known as All Kids Count, which began in 1992. The Institute focuses on the use of information technology and informatics to solve complex public health problems. The Institute's mission is to improve the performance of the public health system by advancing practitioners' abilities to strategically manage and apply information systems to address a wide range of complex and emerging public health issues. The Institute's parent organization, the Task Force, was created in 1984 to improve health and human development through facilitating collaborations with a wide range of partners throughout the world. The Task Force works with global and domestic leaders and organizations to address public health needs by creating coalitions, reaching consensus, and leveraging scarce resources in the areas of infectious diseases, informatics, child health and development, and injury control.

The Institute has a legacy of creating successful collaborations to address a broad range of public health needs. The All Kids Count program had a collaborative approach to assisting public health practitioners in developing immunization registries that included designing a learning network as well as small workgroups that produced knowledge products. The Institute's collaborative approach extends to learning models, and the CoP has emerged as a viable knowledge management tool that helps practitioners meet their knowledge needs.

About *Connections*

The *Connections* CoP was formally recognized in June 2001 at a landmark meeting in Atlanta, Georgia. *Connections* evolved from the work of the All Kids Count program (1992–2000), one of the first large-scale public health informatics initiatives involving electronic linkage of multiple health sector parties in the U.S. Funded by the Robert Wood Johnson Foundation (RWJF), All Kids Count focused on assisting state and local health departments in developing immunization registries for the purpose of improving the immunization status of infants and preschoolers across the nation. In 2000, the Institute broadened its focus to include integration efforts among immunization registries with other early child health information systems.

Integrated child health information systems share individual health data across public health programs, with clinical care providers in the community, hospitals, laboratories, and other entities that need the information to provide appropriate care and services to an individual child. Public health agencies are responsible for tracking a child's immunization history, newborn hearing, and dried blood spot screening, as well as for providing nutritional counseling when appropriate. From a public health perspective, the intent of integrating these information systems is to provide to the child's physicians and other care providers a consolidated, comprehensive record of all services and care a child has received. Authorized users can electronically access a child's record and determine his or her care history, as well as what services a child needs now, i.e., immunization, lead screening, or hearing screening. Currently, child health information is fragmented and often not timely. This leaves the potential for children to miss important health care and social services.

There are many challenges impeding the integration of these systems. Most health departments are organized into program-specific or disease-specific silos, each with its own information system that is frequently not interoperable. Funding for child health programs comes to the health department most often via federal agencies. These agencies perpetuate the fragmented organization of the health department by providing little funding to organization-wide infrastructure, such as information systems. There are few standards in place for guiding the development and electronic linkages of these systems. In essence, the challenges to integrating information systems within health departments are organizational, economic, and, to a lesser degree, technical.

As the Institute began its work in the integrated child health arena, we talked to many public health practitioners, including Rhoda Nicholas, about the challenges to integration. The Institute sought ideas on how to move the nation forward in bringing these systems and people together for the health of our nation's children. All of the practitioners we spoke to noted the importance of learning from one another and participating in a forum within which they could collaborate and address these complex challenges. Building on the Institute's historical knowledge of facilitating coalitions and collaboration, the genesis of forming a CoP took root, and *Connections* was launched.

The *Connections* CoP is facilitated as a peer-to-peer learning community based on the work and theory of social learning networks.[1] *Connections* seeks to maximize interactions among members to promote learning. Members work collaboratively to produce knowledge artifacts that can influence the development of integrating early child health information systems to serve public health practitioners and their stakeholders.

The community has described its intent by focusing on three activities. These are:

- To identify gaps and barriers in knowledge needed to develop integrated systems, and to develop strategies, products, and activities to mitigate or to address the identified obstacles.
- To identify best practices in the development of integrated child health information systems to address issues of policy, leadership, funding, governance, and collaboration, in addition to the potential technical solutions that lead to improved health outcomes.
- To disseminate materials, products, and practices that are developed by the community to the broader audiences of public health, clinical providers, and other interested parties.

Current community membership is made up of public health practitioners from more than twenty-one states and New York City. The vast majority of members are employed by public health departments. Members of *Connections* may have program management, information technology, or leadership roles in public health. A few members are consultants to public health department staff, and membership is open to anyone with an interest in integrating child health information systems. While RWJF funded the initiation of *Connections* through 2004, it is currently being funded by the Health Resources and Services Administration, Maternal and Child Health Bureau (HRSA/MCHB).

Creating a Community

In launching *Connections*, the Institute researched communities of practice to design a community that would be successful in assisting public health practitioners in their efforts to develop integrated child health information systems. The Institute defined the following five principles in governing the community:

1. **Use members' time wisely.** We do this by facilitating meetings with the goal of providing value in every discussion. We understand that our face-to-face time is limited, and members' time is valuable.
2. **Communicate continuously.** The Institute creates a communication loop in which knowledge gained and lessons learned are immediately fed back to the members. We use a combination of online and printed resources to provide summaries and share resources.
3. **Engage thought leaders.** We seek and encourage involvement from innovative public health practitioners who can share examples of challenges and successes. This benefits the members and helps disseminate knowledge and encourage innovation throughout the public health community.
4. **Incorporate quality management.** We focus on members as customers, seeking member involvement in products and activities, measuring the value of the CoP to the members, rewarding leadership among the membership, and seeking ways to improve our methodology for facilitating and guiding the CoP.
5. **Create member ownership of the community.** We encourage the community to mold the activities and tasks within the community by soliciting member input into meeting design, and engaging members to identify topics of interest for learning opportunities and in planning community activities.

Since there were few written guidelines on how to approach integration within the public health environment, face-to-face interactions where members could learn from each other's experience became strategically important. However, the Institute also wanted to take full advantage of technology and created a virtual space for members to collaborate. ConnectionsZone is an interactive Web site that allows for threaded discussions, document sharing, and development. Monthly conference calls are facilitated that highlight experts who address a community challenge, and electronic newsletters are sent to members and other child health information system stakeholders.

The Institute and the CoP have been very fortunate to receive funding from two sponsors to support the facilitation, management, and activities of *Connections.* The sponsorship of the CoP has supported the attendance of members in face-to-face meetings and workgroups by providing reimbursement of travel costs. In addition, these funds are used to provide staff support to the community, to fund the development of knowledge artifacts, and engage subject matter experts and consultants for the development of specific work products.

Funding sources have impacted the Institute's approach to facilitating the CoP. Private philanthropic support is more flexible, and has allowed for a wider range of activities among members. Typically, government sources of funding are often restricted to a very narrow focus, which may require greater flexibility on the part of the community members and facilitators to negotiate mutually beneficial goals, activities, and projects.

Throughout the history of *Connections*, the members have routinely identified the most urgent issues on which they would like to collaborate—those that could lead to the development of approaches or guidelines that would have an impact. The Institute creates workgroups of members, facilitates the development of the knowledge artifacts, and disseminates them to all interested stakeholders (Table 11.1).

The face-to-face interactions are by far the most valued activity within *Connections*—both the community-wide meetings and the smaller workgroup meetings. The community-wide meetings are conducted at a member's site and are often called site visits. Members are given an opportunity to visit colleagues for an in-depth look at the various aspects of their integration efforts. The site visits are designed by members, for members, and supported by the Institute staff. Members vote to select the host site, and hosting is voluntary.

Once a site has been selected, the Institute staff works closely with the site-visit hosts to support the development of learning opportunities. The meetings are planned to provide multiple opportunities for interaction and reflection. Rather than offering a series of presentations, the agendas are planned to incorporate periods of discussion and opportunities for networking in between the short presentations that are provided by members and stakeholders. Members are often recruited to facilitate roundtable discussions in which the participants are asked to describe how the presented material can be applied to their own situations. Members have

Table 11.1: *Connections* Knowledge Products

Integration of Newborn Screening and Genetic Services Systems: A Sourcebook for Planning and Development
Integration of Newborn Screening and Genetic Services Systems: A Tool for Assessment and Planning
Creating a Road Map: Sharing Knowledge about Integrating Child Health Information Systems Volume One and Two
Journal of Public Health Management and Practice: November 2004 Supplement
The Unique Records Portfolio: A Guide to Resolving Duplicate Records in Health Information Systems
A Framework for Integrating Child Health Information Systems: Principles, Core Functions and Performance Measures
Evaluation Toolkit for Integrated Health Information Systems
Business Case Model: A Technical Tool for Calculating the Benefits and Costs of Integrating Child Health Information Systems
De-duplication Technology and Practices for Integrated Child Health Information Systems

an opportunity to query other participants in informal conversation and dialogue, all as part of the meeting design.

In addition to allowing time during the agenda for deepening inquiry and reflection, meetings are planned with ample unstructured time to allow for the development of relationships between attendees. Breaks are generally at least one half hour, and are seen as a critical element of the meeting design. Evaluation of the *Connections* community has documented the value of the relationships members create at the meetings, relationships that sustain the sense of community over time and in between meetings. In addition to the frequent and longer-than-usual breaks, social networking opportunities are provided in the evening. The intentional focus on opportunities to create and sustain contact with other members of the community through face time is one element of meeting design that may not occur in typical conference planning.

The site visits have proven to be the "engine of information sharing," as noted by our evaluators. The most valuable aspect of these meetings seems to be when the hosts present their work. In our experience with *Connections*, members learn most and feel engaged when there is a sufficient level of trust for the exchange of war stories, failures, and lessons learned. We view the site visits as an essential aspect of the success and longevity of this particular community.

Evaluating *Connections*

To create the most valuable community for the members, the Institute engages in continuous process evaluation along with a more comprehensive outcome evaluation. We have built evaluation and feedback mechanisms into community activities, with a special focus on the face-to-face meeting events. We use both quantitative and qualitative methods in evaluating these events. In 2003, the Institute conducted a comprehensive outcome evaluation of *Connections*.

Process Evaluation

In evaluating the community-wide meeting, the Institute uses a two-pronged approach, conducting onsite post-evaluation for the meetings, as well as post-activity focus group interviews. To provide a more objective assessment of the meetings, we have hired external consultants, Silver Creek Associates, to design and conduct the focus group interviews to consider what worked and what did not. The Institute provides the consultants with the meeting participant list. They randomly select meeting participants for the post-meeting focus groups. If the Institute tried a new activity at the meeting, the facilitator's guide would be designed to strategically capture feedback on the new activity. Silver Creek Associates also interviews community members who did not participate in the community meeting to capture possible barriers to participation. Information from these evaluations directly impacts the design of the next community meeting.

To capture the exchange of information between members at the meetings, the Institute engages the attendees in a "get-and-give card" activity. We provide these cards—the get card on separate colored stock paper from the give card—at the meetings, and encourage the members to write down when they have *received* information or artifacts from another member, as well as when they have *given* advice or artifacts. We document these interactions for two reasons. First, to help guide our design of meetings and conference calls. If we see a theme or a specific issue mentioned several times in the cards, we know that this is a priority issue for the community that we might help the community address. Second, this documentation is another method for helping the sponsors to understand the value that the members derive from participating in the community. Many of the workings within a community are invisible to the casual observer, and tangible results often are difficult to document. The get-and-give card approach allows for the documentation of individual personal exchanges of information that would otherwise go unnoticed in most instances.

Outcome Evaluation

In 2003, the Institute hired Silver Creek Associates to conduct an extensive community-wide evaluation of *Connections*. Using the Wenger framework[3] for a CoP, Silver Creek Associates developed an evaluation approach that covered the community's practice, membership, and domain.[2] By looking at all three aspects of the community, it sought to determine:

1. Did the members benefit on an individual professional level?
2. Did participating in *Connections* affect the approach of member organizations in planning and managing their information system initiatives?
3. Did participating in *Connections* accelerate the development of the members' integrated information system projects?

Silver Creek used several approaches in conducting the evaluation, including:

■ Individual interviews with members to generate complex narratives and produce hypotheses to be tested.
■ Group conversations to elicit shared experiences among members. Group interviews are ideal for jogging memories.
■ A Web-based survey to provide a quantitative analysis.

Results from this evaluation show that all CoP members, without exception, gained tangible benefits by participating in *Connections*. One member reported that participating in *Connections* reduced by six months the time necessary to develop an integrated child health information system. The community-wide site visits were reported to be the most valuable activity facilitated by the Institute. However, members also reported a lack of energy between the community meetings, including online discussions. They reported that the technology for ConnectionsZone was outdated, slow, and not user friendly. This comprehensive evaluation assisted the Institute in transitioning the community in 2004 when the community faced a change in funders. Knowing that funding would be more limited, the Institute put more emphasis on virtual forums and purchasing a more robust interactive Web site product for ConnectionsZone. We also have studied and implemented strategies for engaging members in online discussions, as well as conference calls and Web seminars.

Lessons Learned

During the past eight years of facilitating *Connections*, there have been plenty of opportunities to learn. Our three most important lessons come from successes and failures, literature research, and observations from other communities of practice. These three lessons are by no means all that we have learned, but are the most important to consider when creating and facilitating a CoP:

1. Do not overmanage a community.
2. Nurture trust.
3. Understand the nature of the knowledge you are seeking to transfer.

Our experience tells us that there are a number of pitfalls to avoid when facilitating a CoP. The first of these is "overmanagement." Too much structure dampens the community energy, innovation, and ownership. The second lesson, "nurture trust," seems obvious on the surface, but the trick is in *how* to nurture the trust. We offer up some strategies that have helped us. Lastly, one needs to understand the different types of knowledge that are being targeted within the community and design the capture of that knowledge according to its type. This is a cautionary measure to those who have decided on the approach to knowledge transfer before really understanding the type of knowledge they are trying to capture.

Do Not Overmanage a Community

The Institute has learned that facilitating a CoP is an art form that requires balance. There is a fine line between providing too much structure versus too little leadership, as well as in balancing the needs of the community with the needs of the sponsor.

As the host organization of the *Connections* CoP, we have been required to consistently negotiate between the needs of members and the needs of sponsors. For example, sponsors often want community members to focus on national priorities.

However, members' learning needs are often far more practical and operationally oriented. There have been times when we have agreed, without consulting the membership, to conduct activities on behalf of the community that were priorities for funders. We have learned that if the activities proposed by the sponsors have no value to the members' practice, the members are unlikely to be enthusiastic about participating. In order to preserve the functioning of the community, we have on one occasion created a separate venue for an activity, upon the insistence of a sponsor, that we believed would negatively affect the community dynamics. Though the Institute has never had to do so, we have contemplated that there might come a time when we might have to turn down funding if we believed that the CoP learning model was not the best approach to meeting the funder's needs. We have learned that when organizations or sponsors impose or prescribe specific activities for the community, members will disengage unless they can see an immediate benefit to their daily work.

Communities of practice operate in much less structured and more organic fashion than do task-oriented teams. Teams often have well-defined goals or an output to be achieved, which serves to coalesce the members. Well-functioning communities seem to establish a rhythm of their own. Development of knowledge moves at a self-defined and self-regulated pace that may or may not meet established business objectives and deadlines. Allowing time for the development of relationships between members is the crucial first step in supporting the natural progression of the community.

Members need to

- Understand each others' expertise *and* problems.
- Gauge other members' reactions.
- Assess their own talents and potential contributions to the community as well as their colleagues.
- Become aware of differing communication styles of members.
- Identify their interests and where their interests intersect with others.[3]

To develop the depth of understanding necessary for the group to work together, facilitators need to design forums in which the strategy deliberately creates room to interact. We have found that holding social evening functions, informal in nature, is less threatening and therefore ideal in assisting the members in "getting to know one another." This process takes time and often is not acknowledged as important, when in fact the value of the CoP will not be fully realized in the absence of these activities.

In short, balancing a variety of needs, providing room for the community to organically grow, yet providing a framework for that growth is the art of facilitating a community. In our experience an overmanaged CoP is likely to morph into some other type of group, which on the surface continues to look like a CoP, but lacks the value of the community in its true sense.

In *The Speed of Trust*, Stephen M.R. Covey identifies the following behaviors in a high-trust organization:

- Information is shared openly
- Mistakes are tolerated and encouraged as a way of learning
- The culture is innovative and creative
- People are loyal to those who are absent
- People talk straight and confront real issues
- There is real communication and real collaboration
- People share credit abundantly
- There are few "meetings after the meetings"
- Transparency is a practiced value
- People are candid and authentic
- There is a high degree of accountability
- There is palpable vitality and energy—people can feel the positive momentum

Reprinted with permission from *The Speed of Trust*, Stephen M.R. Covey

Nurture Trust

Trust is a rare commodity but essential to a healthy and productive community of practice. The challenge is how to nurture trust among the community members as well as between the members and the community facilitator. For *Connections*, we have found that the degree of trust correlates to the number of face-to-face interactions the members have, the environment created within the meetings, and the willingness on our part in being transparent about decisions made on behalf of the community.

In Silver Creek Associates' 2003 evaluation, members reported that the site visits "are not like the usual conferences showcasing best practice"[2] but that these meetings offered much greater depth and opportunity for discussion. In addition, members reported value in statements and questions "made in a spirit of voluntary vulnerability, admitting to being stuck, to having made poor choices, to not knowing and needing help."[2] The evaluation also noted that if one element was to be singled out as contributing to the benefit of participation, it would be the "community culture created, made of safety, trust, valued relationships and commitment to mutual support."[2] Moreover, our experience indicates that cross-organizational interactions allow a nonthreatening dialogue because members do not have to watch their organizational backs.

Trust is one dimension of success that is difficult to measure and often neglected in organizations. Steve Denning, an organizational consultant and author, notes that "trust levels in large organizations are rarely, if ever, sufficiently high enough to support open sharing of knowledge."[4] Trust is a commodity that needs to be nurtured, developed, and intentionally attended to. In community building, we've learned that trust is built through open dialogue, allowing vulnerability, engaged sharing, and transparency—all elements of meeting design.

The development of trust is facilitated in a number of ways. First, there is some level of consistency in the participation in the meetings so that relationships can be formed. This phenomenon has been documented and described as part of the stages of development for communities of practice.[3] For a CoP to truly exist, members must be able to openly express curiosity, doubt, and the need for knowledge. Trust is often the factor that coalesces the members, allowing for deepening expressions of doubt and open inquiry into the "what ifs" that lead to innovation. One way in which the development of trust occurs is through the open inquiry into "what went wrong." In fact, it seems that the "lessons learned" aspect often is the most engaging and popular part of the *Connections* community meetings.

Creating an environment of trust in *Connections* began with the first community-wide site visit meeting in Missouri. A quote from a program evaluation in 2003 led us to understand the importance of that first visit. "The main enabler of information sharing was community safety. Safety means participants can share information without fearing negative consequences, for instance in terms of how they are regarded in the community. The first site visit in Missouri established and confirmed a norm of safety and candor; not everything goes right the first time, mistakes are part of learning, they need to be acknowledged in public for learning to take place and to be shared."[2]

Some members acknowledge how this combination of safety and trust are hard to find in other settings, including at the usual conferences in which best practices are presented.

Understand the Nature of the Knowledge You Seek to Transfer

A key element of knowledge management techniques is identifying appropriate knowledge transfer practices. The site visit model was identified as a viable strategy based on feedback from members, and there is evidence to support its efficacy as a practice. Nancy M. Dixon, author of *Common Knowledge*, has categorized a number of methods of knowledge transfer, describing the need for particular methods based on a combination of factors. The knowledge transfer methodology she identified for complex, nonroutine, strategic issues, such as developing integrated child health information systems and working toward creating interoperability across multiple systems (public health, private providers, specialist's hospitals, laboratories, etc.), is known as "strategic transfer."[5] Successful strategic transfer occurs only with a high degree of personal interaction. The approach used to facilitate *Connections* relies heavily on face-to-face meetings. It is considered the most valuable aspect of the community, where members can find solutions to their problems and discuss challenges.

With the change in funding levels in 2004, an attempt was made to support the community more heavily through technology. A virtual community was established to allow members to connect between site visits. The Institute upgraded the ConnectionZone technology to include chat room, document sharing, and polling capability. Discussion folders were created for hot issues the community faced. Staff members were assigned to facilitate specific issues, thought leaders were designed for threaded discussions, and a consultant was hired as an expert to guide the facilitation of the online community. But we found members did not embrace this approach. Some members reported that there was not enough value in the discussions. Others reported that the technology did not fit in with their daily workflow.

After a year of intense staff effort and resources dedicated to the technology to support the virtual community, a conversation with a member ended the amount of effort focused on this activity. The member called the facilitator and asked, "Why would I use ConnectionsZone when I can just send an e-mail or call someone directly?" Explaining the benefits of documented discussions to other members just was not incentive enough to warrant the change in workflow processes—even when push technology was employed. This was a hard learning experience for the organization, and now we understand why it did not work. We were trying to promote a particular method of transfer that did not fit the situation.

Our first error was in trying to mix keeping in contact and the potential for knowledge transfer to occur. As the member noted, if she wanted to contact someone, she would just e-mail or phone the person she wanted to access. Logging on to a system that required a password was an extra step that had little value. The informal conversations that take place between members are key to developing a community of practice, but the technology of the virtual community was not supporting that contact.

The second element of the virtual community was to serve as a document repository. An important aspect of strategic transfer is one of "sense-making." Dixon describes sense-making as "synthesizing multiple voices." This act of synthesis turns out to be what was missing from the early knowledge management strategies for *Connections*.

Dixon notes that document repositories alone are not effective for strategic transfer for a number of reasons. Strategic transfer is utilized in complex situations, ones in which the act of knowledge transfer occurs infrequently, and is nonroutine. The development of integrated information systems certainly fits this description. In many instances, practitioners were developing completely new methods of information exchange. Problems to be solved arise in areas that touch on issues of policy, personnel, technology, legal, data security, and a host of other elements that create layers of complexity.

One of the valued aspects of participating in *Connections* is to work on common problems in the form of workgroups. Within these forums, we function as the sensemakers, synthesizing information across the members and identifying commonalities that could be documented, described, and created as knowledge artifacts. The knowledge artifacts are then disseminated to the broader public health audience. As Dixon points out in her book, *Common Knowledge*, "knowledge is transferred most effectively when the transfer process fits the knowledge being transferred." Understanding the nature of the domain[3] of the community and the nature of its practice is key to developing knowledge transfer methods that fit the needs of the community.

Conclusion

Facilitating the *Connections* CoP has been full of lessons about the challenges and benefits of CoPs as a knowledge management strategy. Most of all it has been rewarding.

As public health agencies grapple with new partnerships such as health information exchanges, and health challenges such as chronic disease prevention, bioterrorism, and preparedness, communities of practice can be a valuable approach to organizational learning, since no roadmaps exist to guide us in addressing these challenges. Communities of practice provide public health practitioners the opportunity to learn from one another, work together on finding solutions, and share their knowledge with the broader public health community.

Sustaining a CoP based on the *Connections* model, which calls for frequent face-to-face interactions, is a challenge. This model is resource intense in a time when most public health agencies are facing budget shortfalls. Virtual communities may gain increasing popularity as a viable alternative to the model described here. However, our own experience teaches us that technology alone is not a sufficient solution to meet complex knowledge needs. *Connections* has proven that by investing in the community, one leverages resources, and public health practitioners working in the same focus area benefit by not recreating the wheel. Funding evaluation of these entities also can be expensive. As challenging as these activities are, justifying these communities to potential funders is crucial to continued support and in finding new sponsors.

In closing, we wish to acknowledge the current need for leaders in public health to provide an environment that promotes workforce development and innovation to meet the many challenges that we collectively face. Much of the focus of knowledge management emphasizes the capture and dissemination of information, often supported by technological solutions. Communities of practice focus on the knowledge that resides in people. The basic premise of social learning theory is that potential for information to be transformed into knowledge happens in the context of human interaction. For organizational learning strategies to be truly effective, one must appreciate the distinction between information, data, and knowledge,[6] and harness the collective wisdom of the workforce. Our challenge in the coming decades is to extend our learning needs to encompass wisdom, a uniquely human characteristic.

References

1. Lave, J. and E. Wenger. 1991. *Situated Learning. Legitimate Peripheral Participation.* Cambridge, U.K.: University of Cambridge Press.
2. Wild, E.L., P.A. Richmond, L. de Merode, and J.D. Smith. 2004. All Kids Count connections: A community of practice on integrating child health information systems. *J Public Health Man Prac* (November):S61–5. Vol. 10.
3. Wenger, E., R. McDermott, and W. Snyder. 2005. *Cultivating Communities of Practice.* Cambridge, Mass.: Harvard Business School Press.
4. Http://www.stevedenning.com. Accessed Sept. 18, 2008.
5. Dixon, N. 2000. *Common Knowledge: How Companies Thrive by Sharing What They Know.* Cambridge, Mass.: Harvard Business School Press.
6. Ackoff, R.L. 1989. Data to wisdom. *J Applied Syst Anal* 16:3–9.

Chapter 12

The Association of Public Health Laboratories

From Surveys toward Knowledge Management, a Voyage to Cythera

Robert Rej and Neha Desai

Contents

Background

The Association of Public Health Laboratories (APHL) has as its goal to strengthen laboratories serving the public's health and providing information for individual public health laboratories to use in improving their services to the public. By promoting effective programs and public policy, APHL strives to provide public health laboratories with the resources required to protect the health of U.S. residents and to prevent and control disease globally. APHL's core membership is comprised of public health, environmental, and agricultural laboratories. Representatives from federal agencies, nonprofit organizations, corporations, and interested individuals also participate in the association. There is expanding international participation due to the globalization of disease.

Historical Perspective

Although formally constituted under the APHL rubric only in the late 1990s, the association has its origins in a number of antecedent organizations, including the Southern Public Health Laboratory Association (1920s), the State Laboratory Directors Conference (1927), the Conference of State and Provincial Public Health Laboratory Directors (1939), and the Association of State and Territorial Public Health Laboratory Directors (ASTPHLD, 1951). Since its formation in 1946, the Communicable Disease Center (CDC, now Centers for Disease Control and Prevention) has had close interaction with APHL and its predecessors (1).

As befits their historical origins, public health laboratories and APHL remain rooted in areas of infectious diseases and their detection, but many also have expanded to areas of chronic disease, environmental, food, and agriculture testing. There is considerable heterogeneity in the size, scope, and function among public health laboratories. Among the states, size alone varies from about 30 to 1,200 full-time employees; local public health laboratories are likewise dissimilar. Due to this wide diversity, APHL has published recommendations regarding core functions of public health laboratories (2) and has an active research and knowledge management program so that individual laboratories and members can benefit from the experiences and practices of others.

Drivers for Knowledge Management at APHL

Laboratorians are well-known for having written procedures and documentation for laboratory-based activities, usually through standard operating procedures. These are available to new staff and often to other institutions carrying out similar procedures. However, as in many organizations, tacit knowledge often is not captured and preserved to the same degree. This, along with the aging of the laboratory workforce, has led APHL to adopt a knowledge management strategy to capture information ranging from survey data, to lessons learned through experience, to the facilitation of knowledge transfer through training, technical assistance, and consultation.

Areas of Research and Laboratory Support within APHL

APHL supports and advances nine primary areas of public health laboratory activity, and a committee in each area helps guide the association in these major areas. These are listed in Figure 12.1, along with their organization with respect to knowledge management, and summarized here:

Knowledge Management: The APHL Knowledge Management Committee, although formally constituted in 2005, has its origins in activities of the Informatics Committee, which offered expertise in the development of software used to field surveys to members and provide synthesis of acquired data. This eventually evolved into a subcommittee charged with that role, and eventually a free-standing committee: the Data & Information Survey Committee (DISC). Activities were largely involved with APHL surveys of members and laboratories, and review and adoption of APHL policy on data collection and sharing. Considerable numbers of surveys have been mounted by APHL over the past decades, and these provide valuable knowledge of public health laboratory practices (3). However, since surveys often were authored by programmatic areas, there was unavoidable duplication, and changes in methodology prevented optimal tracking of the evolution of the state of public health laboratories. One of the early activities of the Knowledge Management Committee was development of a strategic plan for data and information management, which led to the committee's current structure.

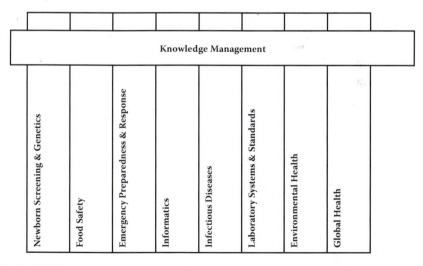

Figure 12.1 Programmatic areas of APHL committees and membership. Not shown are Committees of the Board (Finance, Membership and Recognition, and Annual Meeting Planning Committees) that are not directly driven by laboratory-based areas of effort. Also not shown is the Public Policy Committee, which has a similar liaison structure to Knowledge Management.

The committee and the APHL knowledge management program coordinate the systems and resources to foster the maintenance and sharing of public health research data; provide assistance and guidance in establishing public health forums in order to foster interfaces and interactions among APHL members and stakeholders, and to produce useful and relevant information for public health practices; develop a strategy so that the APHL knowledge management program grows from a data collection and storage function to true information sharing and knowledge management; and help identify the resources that are required to achieve these goals (4).

Organizationally, the Knowledge Management Committee consists of groups of four or five unassigned members and eight members who function as liaisons to the other eight programmatic areas of APHL (Figure 12.1). In this manner, they are able to bring association information on knowledge management practices and resources to their parent committee, but also provide information on program activities back to the Knowledge Management Committee. The eight programmatic areas are:

Newborn screening and genetics: Public health laboratories in each state and territory screen an estimated 4.1 million infants in the Unites States annually for rare, congential disorders. Cumulative data suggest that approximately 5,000 infants are born each year with a health-threatening condition for which screening is currently available. As a public health program, this process is recognized as the largest and most successful health promotion and disease prevention system in the country (5).

Food safety: Each year, foodborne disease accounts for more than 70 million illnesses, 300,000 hospitalizations, and 5,000 deaths in the United States. The potential threat of intentional attacks upon the country's food supply furthers public health concerns. The APHL food safety program collaborates with partners at the CDC, the United States Department of Agriculture, the Food and Drug Administration, and related organizations. The program also works closely with the CDC to support state and local laboratories in PulseNet, the national network of public health laboratories, food laboratories, and regulatory agencies coordinated by the CDC (6).

Emergency preparedness and response: APHL promotes the critical role of public health laboratories in detecting and responding to all health emergencies. In collaboration with the CDC, APHL convenes hands-on workshops to train Laboratory Response Network member laboratories across the country on protocols for detection of bioterrorism agents. It sponsors training to increase the competency of preparedness staff, advocates for resources to sustain key programs, and builds partnerships for a stronger public health system. Its goal is to ensure a nationwide network of safe, state-of-the-art facilities capable of effective emergency response to all hazards and staffed with personnel trained in leading-edge methodologies.

Informatics: Laboratory informatics aims to expedite the exchange of laboratory data via laboratory information systems and electronic data exchange. Public health decisions and patient treatment require the rapid delivery of test results and other public health data. Mounting threats from terrorism, global disease, and natural disasters make the need for near-real-time electronic data exchange even greater.

Infectious diseases: Laboratory detection and confirmation of disease-causing agents by public health laboratories is the cornerstone of effective disease control and prevention efforts. APHL's Infectious Diseases Program promotes the role of the laboratory in disease detection and surveillance, and works to expand and enhance relationships among member laboratories, the CDC, other federal and state agencies, associations, and academia involved in relevant public health activities, including laboratory testing, policy, and training. Working with these partners, APHL develops best practices, guidelines, and training for infectious diagnostic testing in public health laboratories.

Laboratory systems and standards: Guidance to public health laboratories is provided regarding compliance with the federal Clinical Laboratory Improvement Amendments of 1988 (CLIA '88), as well as best practices for laboratory management and improvement. Activities have led to publication and promulgation of the core functions and capabilities of state public health laboratories (2).

Environmental health: APHL's Environmental Health Program focuses on the role of public health laboratories in detecting the presence of contaminants—both in the environment and in human subjects (biomonitoring). Preparing for a chemical terrorism event also has been a priority since the events of September 11, 2001.

Global health: APHL members, who are experienced public health laboratory professionals, are available to work with the program in project countries and to provide training opportunities in U.S. laboratories. APHL provides onsite training programs, equipment procurement, information systems implementation, and laboratory design; technical assistance for strategic planning and program development of laboratory quality assurance systems; and laboratory leadership and management programs for senior and supervisory professionals. Sharing of APHL knowledge with overseas partners is essential.

Knowledge Management Resources

APHL has implemented a number of tools and practices to help foster an environment of knowledge sharing and collaboration among members, member laboratories, committees, and staff. These include:

Listservs: Since e-mail is a comfortable environment and subscribers require only an e-mail client, these have proved to be popular among APHL members. All group membership requires approval by each group's administrator, but activity is otherwise not moderated. Eight Listservs have been established by APHL to foster knowledge sharing; these are equally divided between organizations by function and by discipline (Table 12.1). The first Listserv was established for state laboratory directors in 2001 and is limited to individuals serving in that capacity and allows a far-ranging "private" discussion forum. Similar Listservs have been specifically established for others serving in directorial or coordinating capacities.

Four Listservs address laboratory issues by discipline, or community of interest, and membership is open to all APHL members. These inform and update subscribers of current news and issues directly affecting their laboratory field and allow laboratorians to comfortably exchange information. The newborn screening Listserv started in 2004 and has 128 subscribers representing all fifty states, two territories, and the District of Columbia. Laboratory techniques based on nucleic-acid technology have revolutionized microbiology, and an appropriate Listserv was established in 2007. Quality assurance and quality control issues affect all laboratories and all disciplines and is another area of considerable interest, in particular for following compliance with regulations regarding CLIA '88. In general, these Listservs have been successful at extracting and sharing tacit knowledge among members; however, at present, there is no systematic harvesting or summarizing of discussions. Nonetheless, discussions are monitored by staff, and those with considerable activity are brought to the attention of committee chairs and appropriate staff as potential new work items for preparation of best practice or policy reports.

Wikis: A wiki is a collaboration software tool that allows multiple users to easily create, edit, and link pages together on a Web server. The APHL Informatics Committee has extensively utilized wikis to document the harmonization work being done for the Public Health Laboratory Informatics Program project. The wiki is being used to document development issues and solutions that have emerged

Table 12.1   APHL Listservs

Function Oriented:
• State laboratory directors
• Local laboratory directors
• Environmental laboratory directors
• National Laboratory Training Network state training coordinators
Specialty or Discipline Oriented:
• Microbiology and infectious diseases
• Biomonitoring
• Newborn screening
• Quality assurance and quality control

during the process of developing a harmonized vocabulary for sending data to and receiving data from the CDC.

Portals and collaborative tools: Using such tools, organizations can create, relatively easily and economically, document sharing and collaboration sites that are structured to allow for multiauthor document creation and subsequent versioning. At APHL Microsoft SharePoint is being implemented to organize documents for accessibility and efficiency. Nearly all committees have workspaces in SharePoint to allow for document sharing, as well as a central location for document development.

Jams and JADS: A "jam session" usually refers to a massive online dialogue. A democratic process without hierarchy, a jam offers people the opportunity to come together online to present and evaluate ideas on how to solve a focused set of issues, create new visions, and build consensus. JAD (Joint Application Development) is a methodology that involves the end user in the design and development of an application through a succession of collaborative workshops called JAD sessions. JAD sessions have been used by the APHL Informatics Committee in the development of open-source software and the Public Health Laboratory Interoperability Project for electronic data interchange among institutions.

Education: The National Laboratory Training Network (NLTN) is a training system dedicated to improving laboratory practice of public health significance through continuing education. The NLTN has existed for more than twenty years and has been responsible for maintaining the laboratory's knowledge of laboratory practice; it works to keep public health laboratory practice current with technological and procedural advances.

Research Agenda Council process for creation of new knowledge: In 2007 APHL began the process of organizing current data as well creating new knowledge. A taskforce (Research Agenda Council) was convened and an environmental scan conducted. From the environmental scan information collected, the taskforce learned of APHL stakeholders' interest in creating new information. Therefore, in addition to revisiting old data and improving the quality of data collected, the taskforce will seek opportunities to broaden the scope of information created. The taskforce is currently working to identify opportunities by which to investigate questions identified by the organization's stakeholders to create new knowledge.

Summary

APHL has a considerable history of acquiring new knowledge and sharing its findings with the public health community; for example, substantial data in the Public Health Workforce Enumeration 2000 (7) has been extracted from APHL's consolidated annual reports. Using improved collaborative and knowledge management techniques introduced in the early 2000s along with an improved survey process, the organization is poised to better serve laboratorians in public health in the future.

References

1. Association of Public Health Laboratories. 2002. *Fiftieth Anniversary: Look Back— Looking Forward.* Silver Spring, Md.: APHL. Available at http://www.aphl.org/ AboutAPHL/publications/Documents/Fiftieth_Anniversary.pdf.
2. Witt-Kushner, J., et al. 2002. Core functions and capabilities of state public health laboratories—A report of the Association of Public Health Laboratories. *Morb Mortal Wkly Rep* 51:1–8.
3. Inhorn, S.L., et al. 2006. A comprehensive laboratory services survey of state public health laboratories. *J Pub Health Man Prac* 12:514–21.
4. Association of Public Health Laboratories. 2009. *Knowledge Management for Public Health Laboratories: What, Why & How.* Silver Spring, Md.: APHL. Available at http:// www.aphl.org/aphlprograms/research/knowmanage/pages/default.aspx.
5. U.S. Department of Health & Human Services, Health Resources and Services Administration, Maternal and Child Health Bureau. 2005. Newborn screening: Toward a uniform screening panel and system. Executive summary. Available at ftp:// ftp.hrsa.gov/mchb/genetics/screeningdraftsummary.pdf.
6. U.S. Centers for Disease Control and Prevention. What is PulseNet? Available at http://www.cdc.gov/PULSENET/whatis.htm. Accessed in December 2008.
7. U.S. Department of Health & Human Services, Health Resources and Services Administration, Bureau of Health Professions, National Center for Health Workforce Information and Analysis. 2000. Public Health Workforce Enumeration 2000. Available at http://www.cumc.columbia.edu/dept/nursing/chphsr/pdf/enum2000.pdf.

Index